Handbook of Basic Vascular and Interventional Radiology

Handbook of Basic Vascular and Interventional Radiology

Edited by

Ray Dyer, M.D.

Professor and Vice Chairman
Department of Radiology
Bowman Gray School of Medicine of Wake Forest University
Winston-Salem, North Carolina

Churchill Livingstone
New York, Edinburgh, London, Melbourne, Tokyo

Library of Congress Cataloging-in-Publication Data

Handbook of basic vascular and interventional radiology / edited by
  Ray Dyer.
        p. cm.
  Includes bibliographical references and index.
  ISBN 0-443-08840-3
  1. Angiography—Handbooks, manuals, etc. 2. Blood-vessels-
-Interventional radiology—Handbooks, manuals, etc. I. Dyer, Ray.
  [DNLM: 1. Radiography, Interventional—handbooks. 2. Vascular
Diseases—radiography—handbooks. 3. Vascular Diseases-therapy-
-handbooks. WG 39 H2352]
RC691.6.A53H35 1992
616.1'307572—dc20
DNLM/DLC
for Library of Congress   92-49946
                                              CIP

© **Churchill Livingstone Inc. 1993**

Distributed in the United Kingdom by Churchill Livingstone, Robert Stevenson House,
1–3 Baxter's Place, Leith Walk, Edinburgh EH1 3AF, and by associated companies, branches,
and representatives throughout the world.

Accurate indications, adverse reactions, and dosage schedules for drugs are provided in this
book, but it is possible that they may change. The reader is urged to review the package
information data of the manufacturers of the medications mentioned.

Acquisitions Editor: *Robert A. Hurley*
Copy Editor: *Elizabeth Bowman-Schulman*
Production Designer: *Maryann King*
Production Supervisor: *Jeanine Furino*

Printed in the United States of America

First published in 1993   7 6 5 4 3 2 1

To my loving wife, Susanna,
my sons, Chris and Richard,
and my family, who provided
the impetus, support,
and patience necessary for the
completion of this work.

Contributors

Vincent J. D'Souza, M.D.
Associate Professor, Cardiovascular/Interventional Radiology Section, Department of Radiology, Bowman Gray School of Medicine of Wake Forest University, Winston-Salem, North Carolina

Ray Dyer, M.D.
Professor and Vice Chairman, Department of Radiology, Bowman Gray School of Medicine of Wake Forest University, Winston-Salem, North Carolina

Augustin G. Formanek, M.D.
Professor Emeritus, Cardiovascular/Interventional Radiology Section, Department of Radiology, Bowman Gray School of Medicine of Wake Forest University, Winston-Salem, North Carolina

William P. Jones, M.D.
Staff Radiologist, West Florida Regional Hospital, Pensacola, Florida; Former Fellow, Vascular/Interventional Radiology Section, Department of Radiology, Bowman Gray School of Medicine of Wake Forest University, Winston-Salem, North Carolina

Kerry M. Link, M.D.
Associate Professor and Director, Cardiac Radiology Division, Department of Radiology, Bowman Gray School of Medicine of Wake Forest University, Winston-Salem, North Carolina

William D. Routh, M.D.
Assistant Professor and Director, Cardiovascular/Interventional Radiology Section, Department of Radiology, Bowman Gray School of Medicine of Wake Forest University, Winston-Salem, North Carolina

Mark A. Yap, M.D.
Staff Radiologist, Radiology Associates of Ocala, Ocala, Florida; Former Fellow, Vascular/Interventional Radiology Section, Department of Radiology, Bowman Gray School of Medicine of Wake Forest University, Winston-Salem, North Carolina

Ronald J. Zagoria, M.D.
Associate Professor and Director, Uroradiology Division, Department of Radiology, Bowman Gray School of Medicine of Wake Forest University, Winston-Salem, North Carolina

Preface

The field of vascular and interventional radiology has benefitted greatly from recent technologic advances, as has radiology as a whole. With the increased sophistication and complexity of the procedures, there was an impression that a source of basic technical, anatomic, and interpretive information for this field was not available. Herein lies the impetus for this handbook.

The introductory chapters provide an approach to the patient, information basic to the performance of interventional and vascular procedures, and a discussion of procedural complications. The next group of chapters provides information essential to the performance of arteriography for each major vascular field. Radiographs that reflect the more common indications for these procedures are presented side by side with anatomic line drawings to assist with interpretation. A discussion of vascular and nonvascular interventional procedures follows, and the concluding chapter is a brief overview of drugs useful in the performance of vascular and interventional radiology.

The result is a practical compendium of information essential to the performance of most basic vascular and interventional radiologic procedures and useful in performing those that are more complex. This handbook represents one approach for those early in their training and, by its nature, is incomplete. The information provided represents a common ground from which to start the learning process in this rapidly changing and challenging field.

Ray Dyer, M.D.

Acknowledgments

While the conception of a work belongs to an individual, its reality is a tribute to many. With regard to those who have assisted me in this work, I am blessed. I would like to thank Dr. Douglas Maynard, my chairman, who nurtures the environment where work such as this can be done. I would like to thank my former chairman, Dr. Ted Keats, and my former colleagues, Dr. Wayne Gandee and Dr. Charles Tegtmeyer, all of whom fostered my initial interest in radiology. I also wish to thank my colleagues who contributed to this book and answered each question, knock, ring, and note unselfishly and tirelessly, and others who provided for me the time away from my clinical responsibilities to assure its completion.

Virtually all of our support staff took some part in the production of the manuscript, but special thanks go to Donna S. Garrison, Ph.D., and Mrs. Nancy Ragland for editorial assistance, and to Mrs. Trish Lueder, Mrs. Dee Gilliam, Ms. Julianne Berckman, and Mrs. Betty Metcalf to whom the bulk of the work fell.

The superb line drawings and anatomic renderings are the work of Ms. Annmarie Beery of the Bowman Gray Biomedical Communications Department and my wife, Susanna Dyer, RN, MSN. The scope of this contribution will speak for itself.

Finally, I owe a debt of gratitude to the residents, fellows, and technologists who posed the questions that this book hopes to answer.

Contents

1

Beginning and Ending the Vascular and Interventional Radiologic Procedure

Ray Dyer

Vascular and interventional procedures are unique in the practice of radiology in that they require the integration of technical, radiologic, and clinical skills. Each procedure is initiated with a request for performance, and it is at this time that the radiologist assumes the role of consultant. The radiologist and the referring physician should begin a dialogue that includes the indications for the study, information to be obtained or therapy to be rendered, and facts concerning the patient's condition that would alter the study's routine performance.

A preprocedural visit and evaluation should then be made by a radiology physician directly involved in the performance of the procedure. Elements to be included in this evaluation are a discussion of the procedure with the patient, physical examination pertinent to the performance of the procedure, and an assessment through history and chart review of factors that would place the patient at increased risk.

A direct, interactive patient–physician discussion of the reason for the procedure, the associated risks and benefits, alternatives to the procedure, and in some cases the risk of not performing the procedure serves the dual purpose of establishing patient–physician rapport and satisfying the elements of informed consent, which must be obtained for invasive procedures. The extent to which potential complications must be disclosed depends in large part upon the legal precedent established in the physician's locale. In some instances, it is necessary only to disclose information similar to that which other physicians in the same circumstances would disclose (reasonable-physician standard). In other locales, the patient's role in the decision-making process is considered paramount, and disclosure must be sufficient to allow the patient to make an informed decision (reasonable-patient standard). The latter model implies that the discussion is more inclusive. As a general guideline, risks that are enhanced by the patient's history or condition, as well as those that are well-established or that may produce severe impairment or death, even though remote, should be discussed and the discussion documented.

Table 1-1. Important History and Physical Factors Influencing Study Performance

Patient condition (unable to lie flat, uncooperative, unstable, intubated)
Status of pulses (determines route of entry)
Coagulopathy (increases risk of bleeding complications)
Uncontrolled high blood pressure (increases risk of bleeding complications)
Dehydration or renal insufficiency, especially if associated with diabetes mellitus (heightens risk of contrast nephrotoxicity)
Asthma or allergy, especially a history of previous reaction to contrast exposure (heightens risk of contrast reaction)
Anticipated entry of obstructed system as indicated by renal failure or jaundice (risk of sepsis)
History of myocardial infarction or stroke (indicates diffuse vascular disease)
Drugs (especially anticoagulants)
Arrhythmia (may be augmented by certain procedures)
Confounding study (recent enteric or large volume intravascular contrast study)
Sickle cell disease (increases risk of vascular thrombosis)
Pheochromocytoma (risk of procedure-induced hypertensive crisis)

Physical examination relevant to the anticipated study should be performed by the radiologic consultant. For vascular procedures, the presence of pulses and their relative strength at the usual sites of vascular entry and distal to these points is critical in determining access and in monitoring therapeutic or complication outcome. Complicating features or a need for expansion of the requested procedure may also be discovered. Responsibility for complications related to the vascular and interventional procedure falls directly to the performing physician; therefore, the physical examination should not be left to the referring physician.

History and chart review are essential to determine factors that may increase the patient's risks for undergoing a procedure (Table 1-1). A history of drug allergy, especially involving previous exposure to contrast agents, should be sought. The need for alternative procedures or pretreatment in the case of previous contrast reactions should be noted. Conditions that increase the patient's risk of contrast injury, such as heart disease, preexisting renal failure, and diabetes mellitus, should be considered. Entry into an obstructed biliary or urinary system with complicating infection increases the risk of sepsis and may therefore warrant prophylactic antibiotic therapy.

The coagulation status of the patient should be assessed, and points in the history or laboratory data suggesting coagulation dysfunction should be addressed. True coagulation defects should be corrected, if possible, prior to the procedure (Table 1-2). Routine vascular studies are considered minimally invasive, but because most complications relate to bleeding, a coagulation panel is warranted. Coagulation assessment is also indicated when visceral transit by anything larger than a 22-gauge needle is anticipated.

The visit and assessment should then be documented in the patient's medical chart. Each element should be cited, including the study to be performed and its indications, as well as factors increasing the patient's risk. Pertinent laboratory data, including that which reflects the patient's coagulation status and renal function, as well as any that may become pertinent, such as hemoglobin, hematocrit, and white blood cell count, should also be noted. The presence and strength of pulses for vascular procedures can be presented in tabular form or noted adjacent to a stick figure for quick reference. Absent pulses or the presence of such complicating factors as grafts or aneurysms should be clearly noted. A plan addressing specific problems, including correction of coagulation abnormalities, the need for preprocedural hydration for those at risk for contrast-induced renal injury, steroid pretreatment, or prophylactic antibiotics, should be developed. Documentation of the discussion of the risks and the fact that consent has been obtained should be included.

Table 1-2. Coagulation Assessment

1. Primary hemostasis—a *platelet* function
   150,000–450,000 platelets/mm^3—normal.
   50,000–100,000 platelets/mm^3 may bleed after severe trauma.
   <50,000 platelets/mm^3 may develop cutaneous ecchymosis after minor trauma. This represents the low end of that necessary for adequate hemostasis.
   10,000–20,000 platelets/mm^3 has risk of spontaneous hemorrhage.
   Thrombocytopenia is corrected to >100,000 platelets/mm^3 before the procedure, if possible, with platelet transfusion.
2. Secondary hemostasis—a result of fibrin formation by intrinsic (assessed by PTT) and extrinsic (assessed by PT) coagulation pathways.
   prolongation of PTT by >30% of normal or PT of >15 s should be investigated.
   Coagulation can be improved urgently with fresh frozen plasma.
3. Drugs
   Heparin—can be reversed with protamine sulfate urgently (1 mg protamine sulfate reverses 100 units heparin).
   Coumadin—can be reversed with Vitamin K but requires 6 h. Fresh frozen plasma can be given to normalize coagulation more rapidly.
   Aspirin—disturbs platelet aggregation. Normalization of platelet function may require 3–10 days following last dose.

Abbreviations: PTT, partial thromboplastin time; PT, prothrombin time.

Preprocedural orders (Table 1-3) should make it clear that an invasive procedure has been scheduled, to preclude the performance of confounding procedures such as those requiring enteric or intravascular contrast material, or those that would place the patient in an unmonitored situation following the procedure. The necessity for preparing possible vascular entry sites and fulfilling special needs should also be addressed. It is generally advisable for the patient to remain on clear liquids, but oral medications can be continued. If the patient is dehydrated or otherwise at risk for contrast-induced renal injury, intravenous hydration beginning at least 8 hours prior to the procedure is suggested.

Postprocedural care is determined by the nature of the vascular or interventional procedure performed. Standard orders for postprocedural care for routine vascular procedures (Table 1-4) should include a statement indicating the type of study performed and the site of entry. Vital signs, the entry site, and pulses distal to the site of entry should be monitored frequently. Bed rest is required, and the appropriate extremity should be at rest for a period of time commensurate with vascular entry size. Entry through a large flow vessel with a small-bore (4 to 5 Fr) catheter, with uncomplicated hemostasis following the procedure, may require observation for 4 hours or less, possibly in an outpatient setting. A

Table 1-3. Preprocedural Orders

Patient scheduled for (*procedure*) in Radiology at (*approximate time*)
Shave and prep (*appropriate vascular entry site[s]*)
Clear liquids beginning 4 h prior to examination
Send chart and orders with patient
Have patient void on call to Radiology
Obtain following laboratory studies: PT, PTT, platelet count, blood urea nitrogen, creatinine, and if appropriate, hemoglobin and hematocrit
Consider:
    Preprocedural hydration (at risk for development of or in presence of renal failure)
    Preprocedural antibiotics (entry of an obstructed visceral system or with clinical signs of infection in system to be entered)
    Preprocedural coagulation evaluation (as indicated by history or coagulation panel abnormalities)
    Preprocedural contrast reaction prophylaxis

Abbreviations: PT = prothrombin time; PTT = partial thromboplastin time.

Table 1-4. Postprocedural Orders

Patient status post (*procedure*)
Condition _____
Bed rest with (*side and position*) extremity at rest for (*appropriate time*) h
Check entry site and pulses distal to entry q 15 min × 4, q 30 min × 4, q 1 h × 2, then q 4 h
Notify (*appropriate person and telephone number*) of bleeding, change in distal pulses or extremity appear-
    ance, or other complications
Check vital signs q 15 min × 4, q 30 min × 4, then q 1 h × 2, then per admission orders
Resume previous orders (if appropriate)
Consider:
    Postprocedural hydration
    Postprocedural antibiotics
    Postprocedural monitoring for complications related to bleeding or sepsis
    Postprocedural monitoring for interventional outcome such as tube output (too much, too little, presence
    of blood), ongoing ischemia (thrombolysis), or recurrent bleeding (embolization or pharmacoangiography)

larger-bore entry or a more complicated procedure generally requires a longer period of observation and possibly overnight hospitalization.

At a minimum, a follow-up interview and note documenting the status of the patient should be placed on the chart within 24 hours after the procedure. In uncomplicated vascular studies, the radiologist's involvement concludes at this point. If periprocedural complications have occurred, or if ongoing therapy is rendered, daily patient interaction and a note documenting this interaction are warranted.

For more invasive interventional procedures, a greater degree of responsibility falls to the radiologist. Frequently, the primary clinical service is unfamiliar with complications or maintenance requirements related to the procedure. Following placement of an indwelling catheter, visits at least daily for the first 3 days after the procedure are indicated. Thereafter, visits every 2 days are generally adequate. The radiologist also bears responsibility for arranging routine visits for the maintenance of the catheter and for providing a mechanism for dealing with acute complications such as tube occlusion or dislodgement.

The vascular and interventional radiologist has a unique role in patient care. Though not without risk, the practice can be extraordinarily satisfying. It is incumbent upon the radiologist to assume appropriate responsibility in preprocedural evaluation, procedural performance, and postprocedural follow-up to assure that the patient receives care of the highest quality with minimal risk.

SUGGESTED READINGS

Cohan RH, Dunnick NR, Bashore TM: Treatment of reactions to radiographic contrast material. AJR 151:263, 1988

Lautin EM, Freeman NJ, Schoenfeld AH et al: Radiocontrast-associated renal dysfunction: incidence and risk factors. AJR 157:49, 1991

Reuter SR: An overview of informed consent for radiologists. AJR 148:219, 1987

Rogers WF, Moothart RW: Outpatient arteriography and cardiac catheterization: effective alternatives to inpatient procedures. AJR 144:233, 1985

Silverman SG, Mueller PR, Pfister RC: Hemostatic evaluation before abdominal interventions: an overview and proposal. AJR 154:233, 1990

Spies JB, Rosen RJ, Lebowitz AS: Antibiotic prophylaxis in vascular and interventional radiology: a rational approach. Radiology 166:381, 1988

2

Intravascular Contrast Media and Treatment of Adverse Reactions

Ronald J. Zagoria

CONTRAST AGENTS

Intravascular contrast media can be classified according to their chemical characteristics as either high osmolar or low osmolar. High osmolar agents are ionic solutions of substituted triiodinated benzoic acid associated with a cation. The cation is either sodium or meglumine in proportions varying with different formulations as determined by the manufacturer. For peripheral angiography, media in this class with similar iodine concentrations can be considered equivalent. For arteriography, osmolality of agents in this class is 1,400 to 2,100 mOsm/kg. Low osmolar contrast media have three iodine molecules per osmotically active particle, most of which are nonionic. For media in this class, osmolality is 600 to 900 mOsm/kg. Low osmolar agents cause fewer adverse reactions, produce much less discomfort with intraarterial injection, especially in small vessels such as the distal extremities, and are less toxic than high osmolar agents. For these reasons, low osmolar contrast media have largely replaced older agents for most angiographic procedures.

In 1 to 2% of patients, intravascular injection of low osmolar agents results in adverse reactions, but most of these reactions are minor and self-limited. Minor reactions typically include nausea, vomiting, sneezing, urticaria, pain, dizziness, or headache. Non-life-threatening hypotension, bronchospasm, seizures, and widespread or refractory urticaria are classified as moderate reactions and occur rarely with injections of low osmolar contrast agents. Life-threatening reactions with low osmolar agents can be expected to occur once per 30,000 injections and the mortality rate is one per 170,000 injections. Excluding the sensation of pain, which is markedly reduced in every case with low osmolar agents, the rate of adverse reactions with high osmolar agents is approximately six times that of low osmolar contrast media, although an increased mortality rate remains speculative.

The etiology of these adverse reactions is obscure, and sensitivity testing prior to injection is not a valid predictor of reactions. Some risk factors are known, however. A previous major adverse reaction to contrast media is an important identifiable risk factor, as the repeat reaction rate is 20 to 33% with high osmolar agents. Pretreatment should be

Table 2-1. Management of Patients with History of Previous Major Reaction

Steroids (one of the following):
 Hydrocortisone (Solu-Cortef), 100 mg intravenously or intramuscularly, every 6 h (4 or 5 doses).
 Prednisone, 50 mg by mouth every 6 h (4 or 5 doses).
 Dexamethasone (Decadron), 4 mg by mouth every 6 h (4 or 5 doses).
Diphenhydramine (Benadryl), 50 mg intravenously 10–30 min before ICM injection.
Ephedrine, 25 mg by mouth 30 min before contrast material injection (omit in patients with cardiovascular disease).
Use only low osmolar contrast agents.
Monitor patient closely and maintain venous access throughout examination.

initiated in all patients in this group 18 to 24 hours before contrast material injection (Table 2-1), if possible. Only low osmolar agents should be used for repeat injection in such cases. Age is a risk factor for both elderly patients and patients less than 1 year old. Other known risk factors include renal, cardiovascular, pulmonary, or central nervous system disease, diabetes mellitus, allergies, and asthma. Prophylactic antihistamines (diphenhydramine, 50 mg, orally or intravenously) should be given to patients with multiple allergies. Since the relative risk of acute renal failure is elevated by a factor of 6 in diabetic patients with renal insufficiency, and because patients with renal insufficiency alone also have an increased risk of contrast-induced nephrotoxicity, hydration before and after injection is recommended for these individuals.

TREATMENT OF ADVERSE REACTIONS

With major adverse reactions to intravascular contrast media, the type of reaction determines appropriate treatment. Urticarial reactions are usually self-limited, but widespread or persistent reactions respond to antihistamines (Table 2-2). Vasovagal reactions manifested by hypotension with bradycardia are treated with vigorous intravenous hydration and atropine (Table 2-3). Most severe reactions involve hypotension with tachycardia and some degree of bronchospasm. Epinephrine therapy coupled with vigorous isotonic fluid infusion (Table 2-4) is usually effective in reversing these anaphylactoid reactions. Epinephrine should be administered in small doses to avoid excessive alpha-adrenergic stimulation, which may result in severe hypertension or myocardial ischemia. Attempts should be made to "stay ahead of" hypotensive reactions by early identification and low-dose epinephrine therapy to gradually stabilize and then raise blood pressure.

An H_2 blocker, such as cimetidine, can also be helpful in reversing hypotension, as can corticosteroids given intravenously (Table 2-4). H_1 blockers, such as diphenhydramine, should be used sparingly, as they can exacerbate hypotension when given in large doses.

Table 2-2. Management of Widespread or Prolonged Urticaria

Diphenhydramine (Benadryl), 50 mg intravenously or intramuscularly.
Cimetidine (Tagamet), 300 mg by slow intravenous infusion, or by
 mouth if urticaria persists following diphenhydramine treatment.

Table 2-3. Management of Vasovagal Reactions

Trendelenburg position.
Intravenous normal saline or lactated Ringer's solution as fast as possible.
Atropine, 0.8–1.0 mg by slow intravenous injection.
Repeat atropine injection in 5 min if bradycardia persists (not to exceed 3 mg).

Table 2-4. Management of Major Anaphylactoid Reaction

Assess airway patency, breathing, and hemodynamics.
Begin cardiopulmonary resuscitation, if necessary.
Administer intravenous normal saline or lactated Ringer's solution as fast as possible.
Inject 0.1–0.2 mg epinephrine (1 : 1000 solution) subcutaneously.
If hypotension persists or worsens, inject epinephrine (10 μg/min intravenously) by either of the following
  methods.
    Mix 0.1 mg (0.1 ml of 1 : 1000 solution) in 10 ml normal saline and infuse over 10-min period.
    OR
    Inject 0.1 ml intravenous epinephrine (1 : 10,000 dilution) per min.
Administer oxygen by mask or nasal cannula.
Inject diluted cimetidine (Tagamet), 300 mg by slow intravenous injection over 5–10 min.
Inject hydrocortisone (Solu-Cortef), 200 mg intravenously.
For persistent bronchospasm, administer nebulized bronchiodilator (i.e., metaproterenol). 1–2 inhalations; re-
  peated once after 3–5 min if needed.

Table 2-5. Management of Bronchospasm with Stable Hemodynamics

Oxygen by mask or nasal cannula.
Epinephrine 0.1–0.2 mg (0.1–0.2 ml of 1 : 1000 solution) subcutaneously.
Nebulized beta$_2$-agonist (metaproterenol, albuterol, terbutaline) 1–2 inha-
  lations, repeated once after 3–5 min, if needed.

If bronchospasm is present without hypotension (Table 2-5), low-dose epinephrine therapy alone is usually effective. This therapy can be augmented with nebulized bronchodilator inhalations (albuterol, metaproterenol, or terbutaline) if epinephrine is ineffective in resolving bronchospasm.

SUGGESTED READINGS

Bush WH, Swanson DP: Acute reactions to intravascular contrast media: types, risk factors, recognition, and specific treatment. AJR 157:1153, 1991

Dawson P: Chemotoxicity of contrast media and clinical adverse effects: a review. Invest Radiol 20:S84, 1985

Grassi CJ, Bettmann MA, Finkelstein J, Reagan K: Ioversol: double-blind study of a new low osmolar contrast agent for peripheral and visceral arteriography. Invest Radiol 24:133, 1989

Katayama H: Survey of safety of clinical contrast media. Invest Radiol 25:S7, 1990

Lautin EM, Freeman NJ, Schoenfeld AH et al: Radiocontrast-associated renal dysfunction: incidence and risk factors. AJR 157:49, 1991

3

Basic Angiographic Principles

William D. Routh

PRELIMINARY CONSIDERATIONS

Patient Positioning

The patient's orientation on the angiographic table should maximize the angiographer's access to the arterial entry site, allow adequate fluoroscopic and filming coverage of the vascular territories to be examined, and minimize fluoroscopic exposure to the angiographer during catheter manipulations. Therefore, patient position varies with choice of arterial entry site, type of study, geometry of the room, and design of angiographic equipment.

For femoral artery cannulation in very obese patients, retracting and taping the abdominal panniculus toward the contralateral shoulder and supporting the buttocks on a layer of towels 2 to 3 in. thick will improve access to the groin and make the femoral artery more easily palpable. In infants and small children a "frog leg" position with the hips externally rotated, the feet together, and the buttocks elevated provides optimal access to the femoral artery.

Oblique fluoroscopic and filming projections can be easily obtained with C-arm and U-arm angiographic stands. However, in more conventional angiographic rooms with fixed overhead tubes, the patient must be log-rolled and propped with wedged cushions or be placed on a rotating, cradle-type tabletop attachment for oblique views.

Patient Monitoring

Along with direct visual observation of the patient, continuous electrocardiographic (ECG) monitoring and automated external blood pressure monitoring are performed throughout the procedure in all patients. Pulse oximetry is utilized for patients with significant cardiopulmonary compromise or those requiring heavy sedation. Once an arterial catheter has been introduced, constant intraarterial pressure monitoring can be performed. Monitoring attachments such as ECG leads should be positioned so that they do not impair fluoroscopic visibility during catheter manipulations and are not visible on angiographic films.

Sedation/Anesthesia

In older children and adults, most angiographic exams are performed with only mild sedation. Small incremental intravenous doses of a benzodiazepine (diazepam, midazolam hydrochloride) and/or a narcotic analgesic (morphine sulfate, meperidine hydrochloride, fentanyl citrate) usually suffice. Patients requiring heavy sedation (not easily arousable, with impaired ability to independently and continuously maintain a patent airway) and those requiring general anesthesia are best monitored by an anesthesiologist or nurse anesthetist.

For transfemoral angiography in adults, 1% lidocaine without epinephrine is infiltrated at the entry site subcutaneously and in the deep soft tissues around the femoral artery down to the periosteum of the femoral head. Care is taken not to puncture the artery with the anesthetizing needle to prevent local arterial spasm that may compromise subsequent arterial cannulation. Spasm is of particular concern in children and in transbrachial catheterization.

VESSEL ENTRY

Retrograde Femoral Artery Cannulation

Most angiographic procedures are performed from the retrograde femoral approach (Fig. 3-1). The preferred site of vessel entry is the common femoral artery directly over the femoral head to maximize the effectiveness of manual arterial compression after catheter removal. The entry site must be below the inguinal ligament to reduce the risk of pelvic and/or retroperitoneal hemorrhage since the artery cannot be effectively compressed above this level. An entry site that is too far distal (below the level of the femoral head) also compromises arterial compression and risks entry into the deep femoral artery, making retrograde passage of a guidewire more difficult. In nonobese patients an entry site selected at the inguinal crease will usually be appropriate. If there is any uncertainty as to the level of arterial entry, especially in obese patients, the entry site should be marked fluoroscopically over the inferior aspect of the femoral head.

Both groins are shaved, scrubbed with Betadine solution and alcohol, and sterile drapes are applied, leaving the inguinal area exposed.

Following local lidocaine infiltration a small, full-thickness skin incision is made with a #11 scalpel blade. In children and slender patients with very superficial vessels, care must be taken that the scalpel blade does not contact the artery. The entry site is then spread and the subcutaneous tissues blunt-dissected with a small curved hemostat. For adolescents and adults an 18-gauge modified Cournand needle (Universal Medical Industries, Ballston Spa, NY) is used. For infants and children a 21-gauge needle is usually employed. For right femoral artery cannulation, the angiographer stands at the patient's right side and grasps the needle hub between the right thumb and index finger. The inner stylet should remain fully engaged in the hub with its central fenestration exposed. With the left hand, the femoral pulse is palpated with the index finger just distal to, and the third and fourth fingers just proximal to, the skin entry site. The needle is introduced into the skin site with the bevel up. The needle is slowly advanced at an angle of approximately 45° to the skin surface and in a lateromedial course paralleling that of the common femoral artery. A transmitted pulsation may be felt as the needle contacts the outer arterial wall. With further needle advancement a small jet of blood may be noted through the hub of the hollow stylet. In most cases the needle is then further advanced until it exits the posterior arterial wall and contacts the femoral head (double wall puncture). The needle is then rotated 180°, the stylet removed, and the cannula slowly retracted with both hands stabilized on the patient and the hub of the needle depressed toward the skin. A brisk arterial spurt signals reentry of the cannula tip into the vessel lumen. Holding the cannula stationary with the left hand, the angiographer carefully introduces an appropriate guidewire with the right hand. If the initial attempt at vascular entry is unsuccessful, hemostasis is achieved, if necessary, by brief manual compression, the stylet and cannula are flushed with heparinized saline, and repeat attempts at vessel entry are made. Retrograde left femoral cannulation is best performed with the angiographer standing at the patient's left side and holding the needle in the left hand.

The previously described double wall puncture technique is usually preferred because of its safety and ease of performance. In patients deemed to be at increased risk for puncture site hemorrhage, including patients with poorly controlled hypertension, coagulopathy, or marked obesity, a single wall puncture technique may prevent possible periarterial bleeding from the posterior wall of the vessel.

With the modified Cournand needle, the technique is identical to that described for double wall puncture, except that the fenestrated hub of the hollow stylet must be left uncovered as the needle is slowly advanced to observe closely for arterial return. When this is noted the needle is advanced 2 to 3 mm further to assure that the bevel of the outer cannula has completely entered the vessel. At this point, upon removal of the inner stylet, brisk arterial return should be noted, allowing for guidewire introduction as previously described.

Alternatively, an open, beveled arterial needle may be advanced slowly toward the vessel until brisk arterial return is obtained, at which point guidewire introduction should be possible.

A guidewire with a J configuration of the tip is usually inserted initially. The guidewire is slowly advanced through the cannula, which at this point should be positioned bevel-down to direct the wire tip away from the superficial vessel wall into the lumen. As the wire enters the vessel lumen its J configuration re-forms to provide a blunt, atraumatic leading edge for further guidewire advancement. If any resistance is met, the situation should be assessed fluoroscopically. Forcible attempts to push the guidewire past an obstruction should be avoided because of the risk of vessel dissection. If a sufficient length of the stiff portion of the guidewire has entered the artery, an arterial dilator or endhole catheter can be introduced, keeping the tip distal to the obstructing lesion. Contrast material injected by hand can then be observed fluoroscopically to assess the nature of the obstruction prior to further guidewire manipulation. A stenotic or tortuous iliac artery may prevent passage of the standard J guidewire. In this case, a simple curved catheter such as a JB-1 (Cook, Bloomington, IN) can be used to direct a Bentson wire (Cook, Bloomington, IN) through the site of obstruction. If this is not successful, particularly for more severe or irregular stenoses, a steerable guidewire such as a Glidewire (Medi-tech, Watertown, MA) or TAD wire (Peripheral Systems Group, Mountain View, CA) may be required.

Cannulating the "Pulseless" Femoral Artery

Occasionally it may be necessary to catheterize a femoral artery with a weak or nonpalpable pulse. This situation arises when there is no alternative access for diagnostic angiography or when an interventional procedure (ipsilateral iliac angioplasty) must be performed via this route.

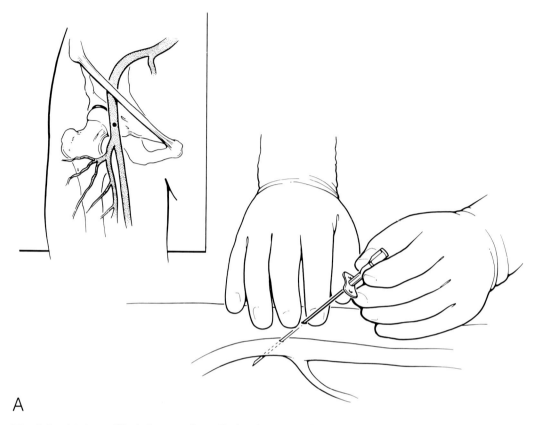

A

Fig. 3-1. (A) A modified Cournand needle is advanced with the bevel up through both walls of the common femoral artery. (*Figure continues.*)

Techniques that may facilitate cannulation of the pulseless femoral artery include the following.

1. The course of the femoral artery is marked on the skin using a hand-held Doppler probe.
2. Intimal calcification of the common femoral artery, if present, is used as a vessel marker for fluoroscopically guided arterial cannulation.
3. In a slender patient with diseased vessels the firmness of the femoral artery may be palpable even in the absence of pulsation, and this can guide needle entry.
4. If the femoral vein can be cannulated and a guidewire advanced into this vessel, fluoroscopically guided needle passes 1 to 2 cm lateral to the guidewire will usually enter the artery.
5. If other arterial access (contralateral femoral or transbrachial catheter placement) has already been established, contrast injection into the distal aorta or appropriate common iliac artery may be used to locate the femoral artery. The use of digital "roadmapping" (see below), if available, is extremely helpful in this situation because it provides a real-time fluoroscopic image of the opacified vessel lumen.

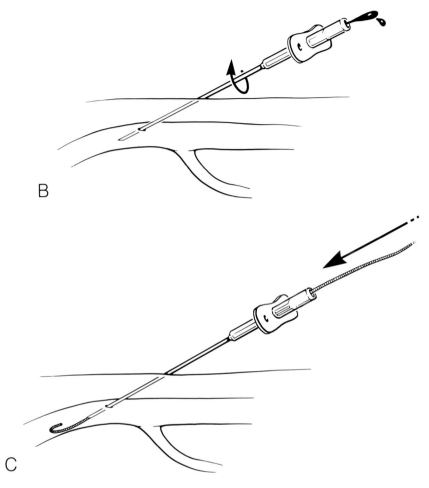

Fig. 3-1 (*Continued*). **(B)** Following the removal of the stylet the needle is slowly retracted with its bevel down until a brisk spurt of arterial blood is noted. The needle is then rotated 180°. **(C)** A J-tipped guidewire is then carefully introduced through the needle into the vessel lumen. Following removal of the angiographic needle, the catheter is introduced over the guidewire.

Antegrade Femoral Artery Cannulation

Antegrade arterial access via the common femoral artery is most often required for infrainguinal vascular intervention (angioplasty, thrombolysis, atherectomy). Catheterization of the superficial femoral artery or a more distal vessel is necessary. The optimal arterial entry site is the proximal most common femoral artery just below the inguinal ligament but well above the femoral artery bifurcation. This technique prevents direct puncture of the deep femoral artery, which may preclude superficial femoral artery catheterization. A skin entry site chosen fluoroscopically over the most superior aspect of the femoral head will usually suffice. If a diagnostic angiogram is available, the level of the inguinal ligament will be indicated by the position of the deep circumflex iliac artery. Antegrade common femoral puncture may not be technically feasible in markedly obese patients.

After local anesthesia administration, skin incision, and blunt dissection, an 18-gauge modified Cournand needle held in the right hand is introduced bevel-up through the skin and slowly advanced at an angle of approximately 45° to the skin surface while the angiographer palpates the femoral pulse with the left hand. The common femoral artery runs in an antegrade direction with a medial to lateral course that becomes relatively less pronounced with advancing age. When the needle contacts the femoral head, it is rotated 180° and then slowly retracted with the stylet removed until a brisk arterial spurt is observed. At this point the appropriate guidewire is introduced (see next chapter).

Antegrade femoral access into either the right or left common femoral artery is usually performed from the left side of the patient with the patient's head to the angiographer's right and the image intensifier to the angiographer's left.

Retrograde Brachial Cannulation

In patients without suitable femoral access, including those with absent femoral pulse, recent nonhealed groin incision, local groin infection, or recently inserted prosthetic vascular graft, the retrograde brachial approach is an alternative for angiographic access. Relative contraindications to this approach include poorly controlled hypertension, obesity, or coagulopathy, all of which increase the risk of puncture site complications.

Evaluation of patients for possible transbrachial arterial access should include palpation of bilateral brachial, radial, and ulnar pulses. Blood pressure should be measured in both arms, and the upper chest and supraclavicular regions should be auscultated for arterial bruits that might indicate unsuspected brachiocephalic occlusive disease that could preclude transbrachial access or make catheterization more difficult.

The left brachial approach is usually preferable for angiographic evaluation of the descending aorta or more distal vessels. The right brachial approach is chosen when there is no other access or when the ascending aorta or innominate, right subclavian, or right vertebral artery must be evaluated from the upper extremity.

A skin entry site should be chosen over the proximal to mid brachial artery at a point where the pulse is easily palpable and the artery readily compressible against the underlying humerus. Too proximal a puncture with axillary artery entry increases the risk of nerve compression injury should local bleeding occur within the axillary neurovascular sheath.

To avoid local vasospasm during administration of local anesthetic for transbrachial arteriography, care should be taken to avoid contact with the artery by the anesthetizing needle. For this reason, infiltration should be confined to the skin and superficial soft tissues only, and deep infiltration is avoided if possible.

Following skin incision and blunt dissection, a modified Cournand needle is advanced parallel to the palpated course of the brachial artery at a 30° to 45° angle to the skin. A spurt of blood through the hub of the stylet indicates arterial entry. For single wall puncture, the needle is advanced a few millimeters more to assure full entry of the beveled tip of the cannula into the vessel lumen. The needle is then rotated 180°, and upon removal of the stylet there should be brisk arterial return, allowing guidewire introduction.

In patients with small brachial arteries and/or a weak brachial pulse, single wall entry can be very challenging, requiring multiple needle passes. The trauma from cannulation of the artery may actually be reduced in such cases by a double wall puncture, which is generally less challenging, technically.

Translumbar Aortic Cannulation

For patients in whom transfemoral or transbrachial access is not available, direct translumbar entry into the aorta is a safe and well-established means of access for aortography (Fig. 3-2). However, selective arterial catheterization or transcatheter intervention is usually not attempted via this route. Since atherosclerotic disease, either occlusive or aneurysmal, usually involves the infrarenal aorta to a greater extent than the suprarenal aorta, a high translumbar approach is preferred. Poorly controlled hypertension and coagulopathy are relative contraindications to translumbar aortography. With the patient in the prone position a skin entry site is selected approximately 6 to 8 cm (four finger breadths) to the left of the midline and 1 to 2 cm inferior to the 12th rib, avoiding the 12th intercostal artery. Following local infiltration of the skin and subcutaneous tissues with 1% lidocaine, a 22-gauge spinal needle is directed under fluoroscopic guidance in a medial/cephalad direction to contact the T12 vertebral body. Additional lidocaine is infiltrated onto bone and along the percutaneous track. Following this same course, a 16-gauge translumbar sheath needle (Cook, Bloomington, IN) is advanced under fluoroscopic guidance to contact

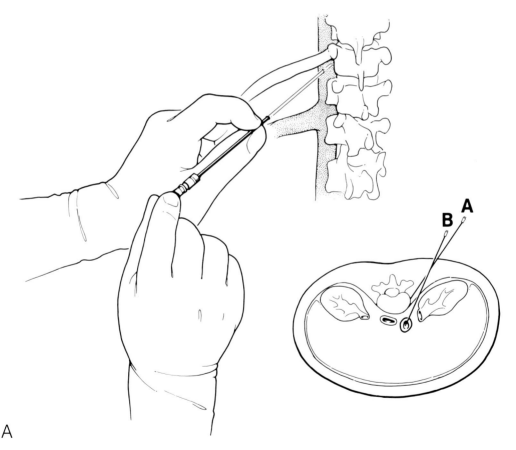

A

Fig. 3-2. (A) A translumbar sheathed needle is advanced adjacent to the left ventral aspect of the T12 vertebral body into the aortic lumen. (*Figure continues.*)

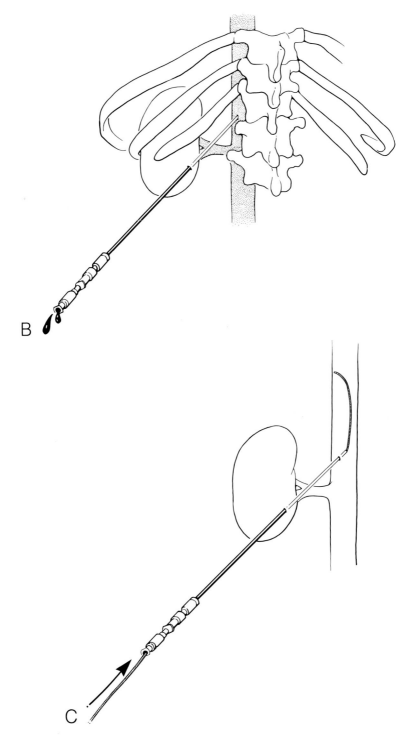

Fig. 3-2 (*Continued*). **(B)** Following removal of the inner stylet, a steady return of arterial blood should be noted. **(C)** A large radius J guidewire is advanced through the stiffening cannula into the distal descending thoracic aorta. (*Figure continues*.)

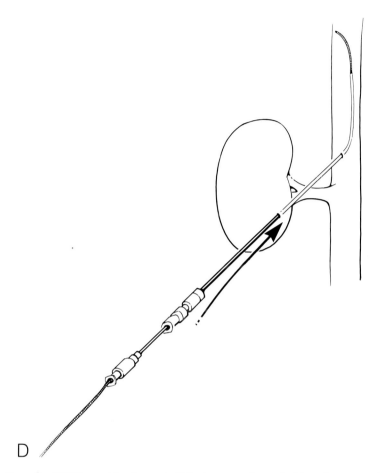

Fig. 3-2 (*Continued*). (**D**) The guidewire and stiffening cannula are held stationary as the outer Teflon sheath is advanced. (*Figure continues.*)

T12. The needle is then retracted several centimeters, redirected a few degrees more ventrally, and readvanced. In this manner the tip of the needle is "walked" along the bone until it just clears the left ventral aspect of the vertebral body. With slow advancement, pulsation of the aorta can often be felt against the needle tip. With further advancement a discrete loss of resistance to needle passage is noted as it enters the aorta. Care should be taken that the needle tip does not cross to the right of the patient's midline to avoid vena caval entry or visceral injury. Once the needle is felt to have entered the aorta, it is advanced a few millimeters further and the pointed inner stylet removed. A steady flow of arterial blood should be observed. Because of the length of the needle, the flow may not be forcibly pulsatile. A large-radius J guidewire is advanced into the aorta and monitored fluoroscopically. While the wire and hollow stiffening cannula are held stationary, the outer Teflon sheath is advanced over the guidewire in a retrograde fashion into the distal descending aorta.

If downstream aortic injection is desired, the guidewire is reintroduced into the aorta and the sheath retracted so that the guidewire can be directed in an antegrade fashion into

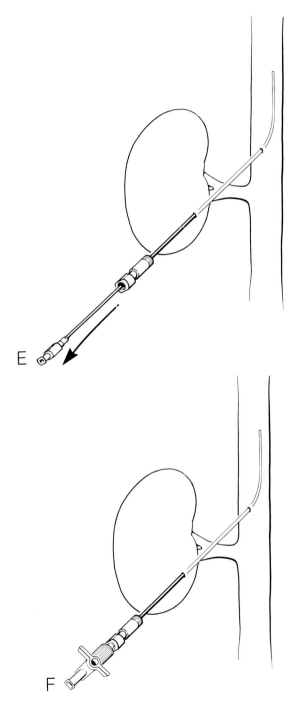

Fig. 3-2. (*Continued*). **(E)** The stiffening cannula is removed, leaving the Teflon sheath in place. **(F)** A stopcock is attached to the Teflon sheath to facilitate flushing and contrast injections.

the infrarenal aorta. At this point the guidewire is stabilized and the sheath advanced distally to the desired position. When retracting the sheath, care must be taken not to withdraw it through the aortic wall so that vascular access is not lost.

Transfemoral Venous Entry

For venous catheterization, a skin entry site is located over the most inferior aspect of the femoral head just medial to the femoral arterial pulse. Administration of local anesthesia, skin incision, and blunt dissection are performed as for arterial entry, except that an attempt to locate the vein by puncture with the anesthetizing needle and aspiration of venous blood may sometimes be appropriate to improve accuracy of venous cannulation. For right femoral venous entry, the right femoral pulse is palpated with the second to fourth fingers of the left hand. An 18-gauge modified Cournand needle is advanced bevel-up at a 45° angle to the skin just medial to the artery. Once the femoral head is contacted, the needle is rotated, the stylet removed, and gentle aspiration applied to the needle as it is slowly retracted. With abrupt aspiration of venous blood, the tubing is disconnected while the needle is held stable and a guidewire is inserted. Performance of a Valsalva maneuver by the patient distends the femoral vein and facilitates venous cannulation and initial guidewire insertion.

If the femoral vein lies deep to the femoral artery, a more medial to lateral needle course may be necessary to avoid passage through the femoral artery. A single wall technique may be employed using an Amplatz (Becton-Dickinson, Franklin Lakes, NJ) sheath needle to avoid transarterial puncture of the vein (Fig. 3-3). This is especially important if large catheters or sheaths are to be introduced, to reduce the risk of puncture site hemorrhage or arteriovenous fistula formation. Steady manual suction is applied with a 10-cc plastic syringe as the Amplatz needle is advanced bevel-up toward the vein. Return of venous blood signals venous entry. The needle is then stabilized and the sheath advanced to its hub. Gentle aspiration is then applied as the sheath is retracted slightly, and when free venous return is again established, a guidewire is introduced.

Arterial Access via Prosthetic Grafts

In patients with existing aortobifemoral bypass grafts, arterial catheterization via one of the femoral limbs of the graft may be preferable to transbrachial or translumbar catheterization. Special attention should be given to thorough preparation and draping of the skin entry site with strict adherence to sterile technique to avoid potential graft infection. A skin site is chosen to assure direct entry into the graft rather than the native artery. In slender patients the infrainguinal course of the graft may be directly palpable. Otherwise a site just inferior to the inguinal ligament and over the area of most pronounced pulsation is chosen. Single wall graft cannulation is attempted with an 18-gauge modified Cournand needle. Should the needle traverse the graft and enter the native artery, passage of the guidewire into the aorta may not be possible because of the usual existence of aortoiliac occlusive disease in such patients. Significant resistance to needle entry into the graft will usually be noted as a result of perigraft fibrosis.

Removal of the Catheter and Care of the Puncture Site

Upon completion of the angiographic procedure and review of the films, unless an indwelling arterial catheter is indicated (e.g., for infusion of vasoactive, thrombolytic, or chemotherapeutic agents), the angiographic catheter is retracted and removed. The punc-

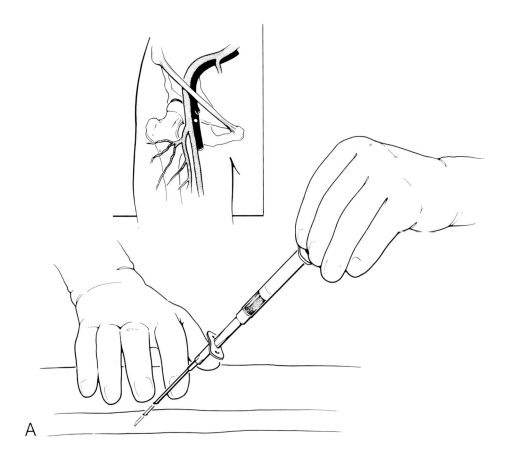

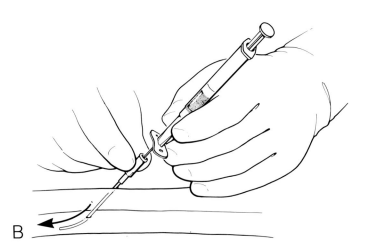

Fig. 3-3. (A) An Amplatz sheath needle is advanced bevel-up while applying steady manual suction with a plastic syringe until free blood return signals venous entry. **(B)** As the needle is held stationary the sheath is advanced into the vein. (*Figure continues.*)

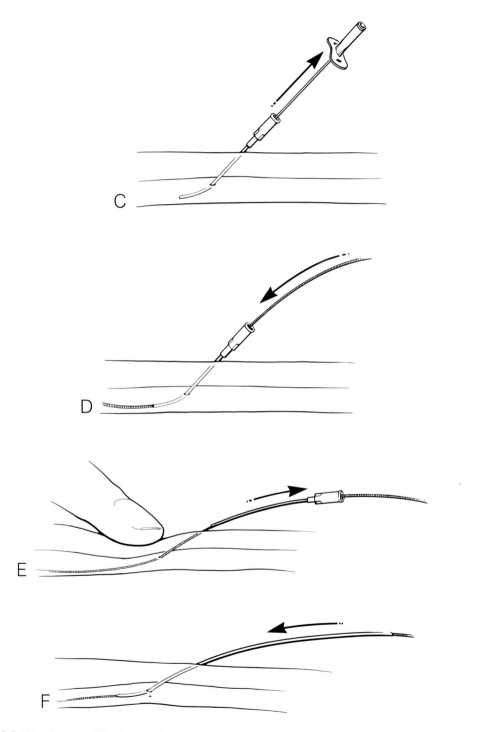

Fig. 3-3 (*Continued*). **(C)** The needle is removed. **(D)** A guidewire is introduced into the vein. **(E)** The entry sight is manually compressed as the sheath is removed. **(F)** A catheter is then introduced over the guidewire.

ture site is then manually compressed to achieve hemostasis. Catheter removal over a guidewire may be indicated, depending upon catheter tip configuration and whether or not a prosthetic graft has been entered (see next chapter).

Before catheter removal the skin entry site should be sufficiently cleared of towels and drapes to facilitate observation of the surrounding soft tissues for signs of a developing hematoma.

For the usual retrograde transfemoral catheter, the index finger is placed directly over, and the third and fourth fingers directly cephalad to the skin entry site. Direct pressure is applied with the gloved finger tips as the catheter is removed. Ideally, sufficient pressure is exerted to prevent bleeding without completely obstructing antegrade arterial flow. Satisfactory hemostasis is usually obtained after 10 to 15 min of compression. Antiseptic ointment and an adhesive bandage are applied to the skin site, followed by application of a compression bandage. The status of distal pulses is established before the patient leaves the angiography suite.

Bleeding that develops during puncture site compression, either externally or as an enlarging hematoma, could be related to or aggravated by one or more of the following factors.

1. Improper compression technique.
2. Improper position of puncture site (too high or too low).
3. Hypertension.
4. Coagulopathy (intrinsic or associated with anticoagulant therapy).
5. Obesity.

Factors 3 and 4 may be correctable by acute pharmacologic intervention (antihypertensive therapy, heparin reversal). Approximately 1% of patients require surgical repair at the arterial entry site because of persistent bleeding, arteriovenous fistula, or pseudoaneurysm formation (see Ch. 5).

TECHNICAL CONSIDERATIONS

A detailed discussion of the technical aspects of film-screen angiography is beyond the scope of this handbook. However, some of the more important technical aspects are reviewed.

Filming Position

Optimal positioning of the patient for filming depends on the vessel to be injected and the probable nature and location of the pathology to be investigated. Generally speaking, during the initial search for an abnormality, maximum coverage of the vascular distribution of the injected vessel is desirable. When a specific area of pathology requires evaluation in more detail, this area of interest should be positioned near the center of the film.

Collimation

As is the case with plain film radiography, proper collimation during film-screen angiography limits exposure to the vascular territory or area of interest and results in reduced patient dose and improved film quality.

Filtration

Discriminate use of differential radiation beam filtration can significantly improve uniformity of film exposure when areas of widely disparate radiation attenuation must be positioned on the same film. Examples include the use of wedge-shaped filters over the lateral abdomen for abdominal aortography and renal and visceral angiography. This produces optimal film density over the central abdomen without excess film density over the flanks. Similarly, wedge filters are essential for performance of high-quality pulmonary angiography to allow adequate retrocardiac exposure without excess film density over the peripheral lung fields.

Radiographic Technique

Mean X-ray beam energy (kVp) should be sufficient to penetrate the area of interest and optimize the radiation absorption of iodinated contrast. Settings from 60 to 80 kVp are usually appropriate for chest and abdominal angiography. Energies above this range, sometimes required for filming of obese patients, may result in substantial reduction in radiographic contrast.

To minimize motion unsharpness and allow for rapid filming rates, exposure times should be kept as short as technically feasible given the constraints of the angiographic system. Thus, to assure sufficient exposure, relatively high (800 to 1,200) mA settings are desirable. These settings are available on newer angiographic systems.

Magnification Angiography

Magnification angiography (increasing patient-film distance with a fixed source-to-image distance) can improve the visibility of subtle small-vessel abnormalities. For example, this technique may be used in examination of vessels in the fingers or for detailed evaluation of peripheral intrarenal arterial branches. To assure maximum detail, multifocal X-ray tubes should be operated at the smallest possible focal spot setting, thus minimizing the penumbra effect, which contributes to image unsharpness. Unfortunately, limited tube heat-loading tolerance may require operation at relatively low mA settings. As a result, to obtain sufficient film density, exposure times must be lengthened, resulting in increased motion unsharpness. This is a particularly difficult problem in obese patients. For abdominal angiography, magnification technique is best suited for slender patients and may actually result in a loss of resolution in obese patients.

Filming Artifacts

To maximize film quality and to avoid obscuring diagnostic information and factitious simulation of pathology, filming artifacts must be avoided. To this end, intensifying screens must be regularly cleaned and ECG leads, intravenous tubing, and contrast-soaked towels and drapes must be compulsively kept out of the field of angiographic view. Metallic tabletop parts also should not appear on films. In clinical situations involving acute trauma or medically unstable patients, angiographic filming may be necessary in spite of superimposed external stabilization or life-support devices. In such cases additional filming projections may be required to circumvent these devices and avoid missing important pathology.

Film Changers and Filming Sequences

Rapid film changers for conventional angiography operate at maximum filming rates of either 4 films/s (Puck, Siemens-Elema AB, Solna, Sweden) or 6 films/s (AOT, Siemens-Elema AB, Solna, Sweden). Moveable floor-mounted stands that incorporate either type of changer are available for anteroposterior or lateral filming using a separate ceiling-mounted X-ray tube (other than the fluoroscopy tube). With this configuration, when changing from fluoroscopy to filming, the table (and patient) must be moved, usually longitudinally, over the film changer. Oblique filming projections necessitate log-rolling the patient or use of a cradle attachment to the tabletop.

With newer C-arm and U-arm systems, a film changer mounted on the fluoroscopy stand adjacent to the image intensifier allows filming to be performed with the patient in the position used for fluoroscopy. The X-ray tube and geometry are also identical. Such systems allow for multiple oblique and cranial-caudal angulations without moving the patient and therefore are especially well-suited for trauma evaluation and interventional angiographic procedures.

The number of films obtained per second and the duration of filming are programmed into the system before each angiographic run. The most important considerations in determining an appropriate filming sequence include the rate of blood flow in the vessel being examined and the nature of the known or suspected vascular abnormality being evaluated. For most situations, multiple film exposures are obtained throughout the arterial phase into the venous phase of contrast flow. Filming rates will generally parallel changes in rate of blood flow; more rapid filming is done during the arterial phase, with slower filming during the capillary and venous phases. The goal is to maximize the diagnostic information obtained during each contrast injection without excessive exposure to the patient or waste of valuable radiographic film.

Representative filming sequences will be given for each of the angiographic procedures discussed in this handbook. These are only guidelines that may need to be modified on a case-by-case basis to best fit the patient and pathology under consideration.

Contrast Injectors—Injection Parameters

A variety of programmable automatic piston-type injection devices are available. These devices provide predictable and reproducible contrast flow rates for angiography. The injector parameters that must be specified and programmed into the system prior to each angiographic run are injection rate (cc/s), total volume of injection (cc), and delay between onset of contrast injection and onset of filming (or vice versa). For a given angiographic examination the parameters are determined both by experience and by an assessment of arterial flow rate as observed fluoroscopically during a hand injection of contrast material. A maximum pressure limit is set to prevent catheter rupture during injection. This limit varies according to type of study and specific characteristics of the catheter (caliber, length, material, side holes). For most catheters, maximum flow rate and pressure are indicated on the packaging label.

An additional parameter called linear rate rise is programmable into most systems. This specifies the time lapse between initial onset and maximum rate of contrast injection. Specifying a rate rise (usually some fraction of a second) may reduce the likelihood that catheter position will be disturbed by catheter recoil during power injection. Catheter recoil can usually be anticipated with smaller caliber catheters lacking side holes, and during large contrast injections. Otherwise, rate rise should usually be set at 0 to optimize vessel opacification for angiography.

Representative contrast injection parameters are given for each of the angiographic procedures discussed in this handbook. These are intended as general guidelines and may need to be modified on a case-by-case basis.

Digital Subtraction Angiography

Digital angiographic systems have evolved to the point that digital subtraction angiography (DSA) may be an acceptable alternative to conventional film screen angiography for a number of indications. Superior contrast resolution of DSA allows for reduction in contrast material concentration and/or injection rate, resulting in reduction in total contrast material dose to the patient. Elimination of scout radiographs and film processing between angiographic runs can significantly reduce procedure time. Digital roadmapping, by providing a real-time fluoroscopic image of the opacified vessel lumen, can be a tremendous aid in guidewire negotiation through tortuous, stenotic, or irregular vessels. This software option is particularly helpful for vascular interventional procedures such as balloon angioplasty.

The quality of digital subtraction images is significantly degraded by motion (uncooperative patient, cardiac activity, respiratory movement, bowel gas motion). This problem is particularly common with abdominal and pulmonary angiography. In addition, limitations in spatial resolution may compromise DSA in the detailed evaluation of subtle small-vessel abnormalities. Limitation of field of view can be a disadvantage of DSA, especially for mesenteric or bilateral lower extremity angiography. Technical innovations that may alleviate some of these deficiencies include higher pixel-density imaging chains that allow increased spatial resolution, larger image receptors for increased field of view, and nonsubtracted digital angiography to limit image degradation by motion.

SUGGESTED READINGS

Grollman JH Jr, Marcus R: Transbrachial arteriography: techniques and complications. Cardiovasc Intervent Radiol 11:32, 1988

Kadir S: Diagnostic Angiography. WB Saunders, Philadelphia, 1986

Lechner G, Jantsch H, Waneck R, Kretschmer G: The relationship between the common femoral artery, the inguinal crease, and the inguinal ligament: a guide to accurate angiographic puncture. Cardiovasc Intervent Radiol 11:165, 1988

Lind LJ, Mushlin PS: Sedation, analgesia, and anesthesia for radiologic procedures. Cardiovasc Intervent Radiol 10:247, 1987

Seldinger SI: Catheter replacement of the needle in percutaneous arteriography: a new technique. Acta Radiol 39:368, 1953

4

Catheters and Guidewires

William D. Routh

CATHETER MATERIALS

Angiographic catheters are available in a variety of materials, including polyethylene, polyurethane, nylon, and Teflon. These materials are rendered relatively radiopaque and therefore fluoroscopically visible by impregnation with barium, bismuth, or lead salts.

Polyethylene catheters are the most widely utilized. They have sufficient stiffness to allow easy arterial insertion and adequate torque control but are still flexible enough to allow selective and superselective positioning. Of the catheter materials available, polyethylene is the most readily reshaped with steam, allowing the angiographer to customize the catheter configuration to facilitate selective catheterization.

Polyurethane has a relatively higher coefficient of friction than do the other materials. As a result, catheter insertion or guidewire passage may be more difficult. A low-friction coating as in the Toray catheter (Toray Industries, Tokyo, Japan) can partially alleviate this problem.

A woven stainless steel wire mesh may be incorporated into the walls of either polyethylene or polyurethane catheters to improve torque responsiveness. The distal segment in such catheters is left unbraided to provide sufficient tip flexibility for selective catheter positioning. However, increased stiffness of the catheter shaft because of the steel braiding may impede passage of the catheter over a guidewire through a tortuous vessel.

Some currently available nylon catheters exhibit an appropriate combination of torque control, relatively low-friction surface, and adequate flexibility for selective and superselective positioning. A good example is the Imager line of catheters (Medi-tech, Watertown, MA). These catheters follow a tortuous course particularly well when used with a hydrophilic-coated low-friction guidewire such as the Glidewire (Medi-tech, Watertown, MA). A disadvantage of nylon catheters, in contrast to those made of polyethylene, is resistance to reshaping with steam.

The low coefficient of friction of Teflon catheters adds to their ease of insertion. However, their relative stiffness and resistance to reshaping limit their usefulness for selective angiography. Occasionally, small (3 Fr) Teflon catheters may be passed coaxially through standard (5 to 6.5 Fr) selective catheters for superselective angiography or pharmacologic infusions. Because of its stiffness and low coefficient of friction, Teflon is particularly suitable for angiographic introducer sheaths and dilators.

CATHETER CALIBER

For any angiographic procedure, the caliber of the catheter must be sufficient to accommodate the contrast material flow rates required for optimal vessel opacification. Caliber selection depends on the rate of blood flow in the injected vessel. In addition, the catheter should transmit the contrast material with a minimum of recoil of the catheter tip to avoid malposition and vessel injury during injection. This is especially important during selective and superselective angiography. For example, a 4 Fr catheter might be capable of transmitting sufficient contrast material to opacify a renal or visceral artery. However, catheter recoil might be so great that a larger caliber catheter is necessary to prevent recoil of the tip into the aorta during the injection.

Occasionally, for superselective catheterization of relatively small arteries, the catheter caliber may be limited by the size of the vessel to be catheterized.

Intuitively, the risk of puncture site complications should increase with increasing catheter caliber. However, within the usual size range of diagnostic angiographic catheters (5 to 7 Fr), this relationship has not clearly been established. Generally, though, the smallest caliber catheter that will not compromise the technical performance or diagnostic quality of the study should be chosen. In pediatric angiography, relatively small catheters (3 to 4 Fr) are routinely used.

CATHETER LENGTH

Obviously, catheters must be long enough to reach from the skin entry site to the vessel being studied. Since the resistance to flow of contrast material varies in direct proportion to the catheter length, excessive length should be avoided. Furthermore, an excessive length of catheter outside the patient makes catheter manipulation more cumbersome.

CATHETER SIDE HOLES

The addition of side holes to angiographic catheters reduces resistance to contrast material injection (increasing maximum injection rate), reduces severity of catheter recoil, and improves distribution of contrast material within the lumen of a large vessel. These benefits are particularly desirable for aortography, pulmonary angiography, and venacavography. Occasionally, additional side holes may be added to an endhole catheter for selective angiography to allow for a sufficient injection rate without excessive recoil and to eliminate the need for a larger caliber catheter. For selective angiography, additional side holes are also sometimes desirable to improve opacification of a proximal arterial side branch.

For selective venous catheterization, especially if blood samples are to be obtained, at least one small side hole near the catheter tip is essential to reduce the tendency for catheter occlusion by the vein wall during attempted aspiration. An important caveat is to avoid passage of embolization coils through a catheter with side holes. Upon reaching the catheter tip, the coil may engage, partially exit, and become trapped in a side hole, effectively occluding the catheter.

CATHETER TIP CONFIGURATIONS

Pigtail Catheters

"Pigtail" catheters (Fig. 4-1) are used primarily for injection of large vessels with relatively high flow rates, such as the aorta, pulmonary artery, and vena cava. The design enables the catheter to remain free in the vessel lumen during injection, to reduce the risk of inadvertent selective catheterization of a small branch vessel by the catheter tip, and to avoid injection of contrast material subintimally into the vessel wall. Multiple side holes in a variety of configurations are added to increase the flow of contrast material and to improve its distribution throughout the vessel lumen. Side holes also decrease catheter recoil and reduce the extent to which the pigtail straightens during the injection.

SELECTIVE ENDHOLE CATHETERS

Rösch Celiac

The simple C-shaped curve of the Rösch Celiac (RC1 and RC2) catheters (Fig. 4-2A & B) is appropriate for most celiac and superior mesenteric angiography. Similarly, this catheter shape is also useful for most renal angiography. Slight manual straightening of the distal catheter tip prior to introduction may improve its conformation to the course of the renal artery.

From the femoral approach, the contralateral common iliac artery is usually catheterized easily with the RC1.

Rösch Inferior Mesenteric

The relatively small radius C-shaped curve of the Rösch Inferior Mesenteric (RIM) catheter (Fig. 4-2C) conforms to the aortic origin of most inferior mesenteric arteries when introduced from the left femoral approach.

Cobra

The tip of the Cobra (C1 or C2) catheter (Fig. 4-2D & E) is relatively easy to direct, and the shape usually engages the renal arteries and the celiac and superior mesenteric arteries. Generally, however, this catheter shape does not conform well to the course of any of these vessels; therefore, for advancement into a stable selective position a leading guidewire is often necessary. Both of these factors increase the likelihood of arterial spasm that could compromise the quality of the examination.

For selective renal vein renin sampling, catheterization can usually be accomplished with a cobra-shaped catheter with distal side holes.

SUPERSELECTIVE VISCERAL CATHETERS

Rösch Left Gastric

The shape of the Rösch Left Gastric (RLG) reversed curve catheter (Fig. 4-3A) must be re-formed, either across the aortic bifurcation or by advancement over a tip-deflector guidewire (see below). The catheter tip is then engaged in the celiac origin, and as the catheter is carefully retracted, the tip advances along the superior wall of the celiac artery

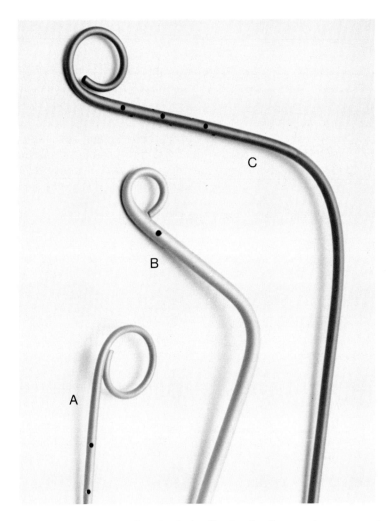

Fig. 4-1. Pigtail-type catheters. **(A)** Standard pigtail; **(B)** Grollman pulmonary catheter; **(C)** Van Aman pulmonary catheter.

and ultimately engages the left gastric orifice. If the origin of the left gastric artery is too far from the celiac origin, the length of the RLG curve may not be sufficient. In this case it may be necessary to fashion a longer-limbed reversed curve catheter with steam.

Rösch Hepatic

Often superselective hepatic artery catheterization can be accomplished by advancement of the simple-curved RC1 catheter over a guidewire. However, when the initial caudal course of the celiac artery is relatively steep, attempts at catheter advancement will produce guidewire buckling and dislodgement. In this situation the tip of the re-formed Rösch Hepatic (RH) (Fig. 4-3B) catheter is engaged in the celiac artery, and as the catheter is retracted its tip advances into the hepatic artery. The orientation of the catheter tip

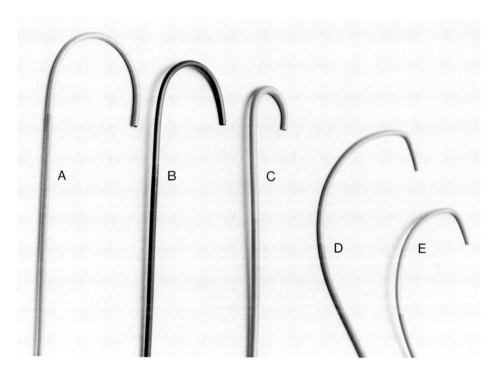

Fig. 4-2. Selective visceral catheters. **(A)** RC1; **(B)** RC2; **(C)** RIM; **(D)** C1; **(E)** C2.

(cephalad or caudad) can be modified by catheter rotation to keep it aligned with the course of the vessel. To avoid vessel injury, a flexible guidewire is often initially advanced into the hepatic artery, and slight traction is maintained on the wire as the catheter is retracted and its tip is advanced into the common hepatic artery.

Rösch Dorsal Pancreatic

The closed distal curve of the Rösch Dorsal Pancreatic (RDP) catheter (Fig. 4-3C) is generally suited to the anatomy of the dorsal pancreatic artery, which usually arises from the proximal celiac artery. Similarly, the gastroduodenal artery can often be catheterized with this shape. A Bentson guidewire (Cook, Bloomington, IN) or an angled Glidewire (Medi-tech, Watertown, MA) may facilitate superselective catheterization of these vessels.

MISCELLANEOUS CATHETER SHAPES

JB-1

The relatively open-angled distal tip makes this catheter shape (Fig. 4-4A) useful for directing guidewires along tortuous or diseased vessels.

Headhunter

The Headhunter (H1) catheter shape (Fig. 4-4B) is used for innominate and subclavian artery catheterization. The catheter is advanced over a J guidewire into the ascending aorta, rotated counterclockwise to direct the tip cephalad, and slowly retracted to engage

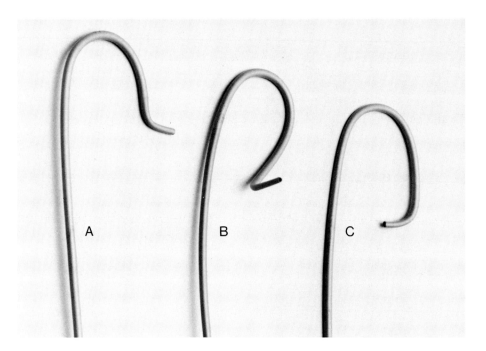

Fig. 4-3. Superselective visceral catheters. **(A)** RLG; **(B)** RH; **(C)** RDP.

the appropriate arch vessel. The catheter is then advanced over a guidewire into the desired position.

Because of the angled tip configuration of the H1, advancement into the brachial artery with contact on the arterial wall may result in localized vasospasm. Therefore, for brachial angiography exchange for a straight catheter should be considered.

In older patients, elongation of the aortic arch may be associated with a much more acute angle of origin of the arch vessels, so that the H1 will not engage their origins. In such cases one of a variety of selective cerebral catheters with more closed distal curves may be used.

Simmons

For abdominal angiography, the Simmons (S1, S2, S3) ("sidewinder") catheter (Fig. 4-4C & D) may occasionally be useful for selective catheterization of aortic branches that arise with a steep caudal angulation. For example, in a patient with a ptotic kidney and a steeply angled renal artery, this catheter may be appropriate. Similarly, right gonadal venography (often indicated in patients with varicoceles) can usually be performed with the Simmons catheter. The S1, with its shorter limb, is preferred for intra-abdominal indications. As with other reversed curve catheters, the shape must be re-formed after introduction either by selective engagement of the catheter tip in an aortic branch, by positioning the catheter over a guidewire across the aortic bifurcation, or by using a tip-deflector guidewire.

Mikaelsson Catheter

The Mikaelsson catheter shape (Fig. 4-4E), which also must be re-formed in the aorta, is designed for selective catheterization of small aortic branches that arise perpendicular to the aortic wall. Examples include intercostal, lumbar, and bronchial arteries. Once the catheter tip engages the vessel orifice, slight retraction advances the tip into a stable position. A Bentson guidewire advanced a few centimeters into the vessel may be helpful in guiding the catheter tip into position, thus preventing vessel injury as the catheter is retracted.

COAXIAL MICROCATHETERS

The recent development of microcatheter systems such as the Tracker-18 (Target Therapeutics, Los Angeles, CA) and its various modifications has made possible extremely selective catheter positioning not previously feasible with more conventional catheter and guidewire systems. This development has been particularly valuable in the field of embolotherapy, especially for neuroradiologic and intra-abdominal indications. The standard Tracker-18 is a highly flexible 3 Fr catheter that tapers distally to 2.2 Fr. A platinum bead incorporated into the tip makes it visible on fluoroscopy. This catheter may be advanced through a very tortuous course in small vessels over a monofilament stainless steel platinum-tipped steerable guidewire. The standard Tracker system is delivered through a coaxial guiding catheter tapered at its distal tip to a diameter no smaller than 0.038 in. Therefore, some 5 Fr and most 6 Fr or larger selective angiographic catheters can be used for this purpose.

RESHAPING CATHETERS

Although a wide variety of preshaped catheter curves are commercially available, the vascular anatomy of an individual patient may require a more customized catheter configuration for successful selective or superselective angiography. For this purpose, a straight polyethylene catheter can be fashioned easily into the desired shape. As a general rule, the shape of the catheter should correspond roughly to the course of the vessel to be catheterized.

The tip of the polyethylene catheter is softened and shaped with steam and then submerged in cool, sterile saline to fix the shape. When very tight catheter curves must be formed, bending the catheter over a flexible guidewire while holding the catheter in the steam flow can help to prevent kinking.

GUIDEWIRES

Angiographic guidewires are required during initial vascular access and may also be used for selective catheter positioning, catheter exchange, negotiation of tortuous, stenotic, or obstructed vessels, deposition of vascular occluding devices, and re-formation of complex catheter configurations. Because a wide variety of guidewires are available, choice of an appropriate wire depends on the angiographer's experience, the study to be performed, and the specific vascular anatomy and pathology exhibited by the individual patient.

Suggested guidewire types are listed, when appropriate, in subsequent chapters dealing with specific angiographic and interventional procedures.

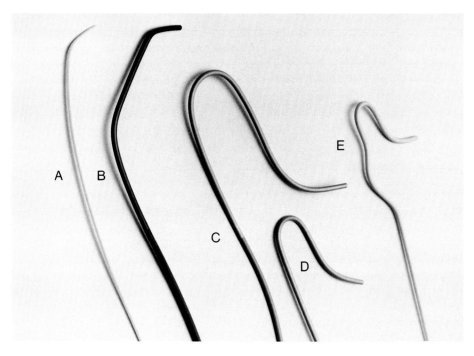

Fig. 4-4. Miscellaneous catheter configurations. **(A)** JB-1; **(B)** H1 ; **(C)** S2; **(D)** S1; **(E)** Mikaelsson.

Conventional "Coil Spring" Guidewires

Conventional angiographic guidewires consist of a long, slender stainless steel coil spring wrapped around a central monofilament stainless steel core. To reduce the risk of guidewire breakage, an additional smaller monofilament guardwire runs within the lumen of the coil spring and is firmly attached to its tip (Fig. 4-5).

In the choice of a conventional guidewire, parameters that must be specified include the following.

1. Caliber—Coil spring wires are available in diameter gradations ranging from 0.018 in. to 0.045 in. To facilitate percutaneous arterial catheter introduction, the guidewire caliber and the nominal diameter of the distal taper of the catheter should closely correspond.
2. Length—For most transfemoral angiographic procedures the guidewire length must simply exceed the catheter length sufficiently to prevent loss of vascular access during catheter placement. Additional guidewire length may be required to exchange the catheter while maintaining guidewire position selectively in a vessel. This maneuver may require a special exchange guidewire available in lengths up to 300 cm. For example, pulmonary angiography can be performed with a 100-cm catheter and a 150-cm guidewire. However, if the catheter must be exchanged without sacrificing selective positioning in a peripheral pulmonary artery branch, a much longer guidewire will be necessary.
3. Tip configuration—The inner core of most conventional guidewires terminates proxi-

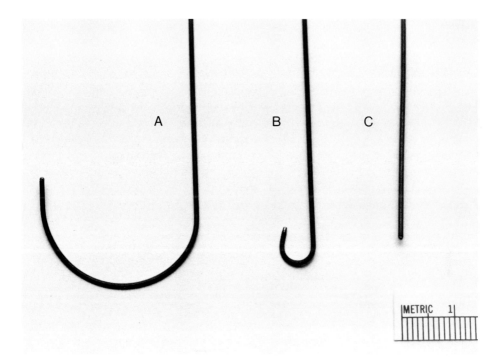

Fig. 4-5. Basic guidewire configurations (0.38 in.). **(A)** 15-mm radius curved J; **(B)** 3-mm radius J; **(C)** straight.

mally to the tip, so that the length of the most distal coil spring is relatively flexible. The tip is then left straight or altered to a J configuration to reduce the risk of vessel trauma even further. The nominal size of the J refers to its radius (with a 2-mm J guidewire the radius of curvature of the distal tip is 2 mm and the diameter 4 mm). To avoid vessel wall trauma the diameter of the J generally should not exceed that of the smallest vessel lumen through which it must pass.

4. Core—The inner core of the guidewire imparts stiffness. When the caliber of the core is fixed all the way to its tip, there is no variation in guidewire stiffness from one end to the other. However, the distal end of the core may be tapered in diameter over a variable length so that the distal end of the guidewire becomes gradually more flexible. The core caliber tapers over a 10-cm segment in a long-tapered (LT) guidewire and over a 15-cm segment in an LLT guidewire.

Graduated guidewire stiffness may aid in catheter advancement along a tortuous course, reducing the likelihood of guidewire buckling.

In a fixed-core guidewire, the core is attached to the outer spring. In moveable-core guidewires, the core is not attached and can therefore be retracted, allowing the angiographer to vary the length of the distal floppy segment.

Special mention should be made of the Bentson guidewire (Cook, Bloomington, IN). This straight, coil spring guidewire has a fixed, tapered core and a particularly long (15-cm) distal floppy segment. As a result, this guidewire is relatively atraumatic when used in small, tortuous, or stenotic vessels. It can also be advanced through reversed curve catheters without disturbing the distal catheter shape.

Heavy-Duty Guidewires

In some situations attempted catheter advancement may be compromised by guidewire buckling. Examples include vessel tortuosity, vessel stenosis, or puncture site scarring, as well as during attempted advancement of a relatively stiff device such as an inferior vena cava filter delivery capsule. Additional guidewire stiffness can be obtained by using a larger caliber wire, if the catheter will accommodate it. Otherwise one of a variety of heavy-duty guidewires may be selected, such as the Amplatz stiff (Cook, Bloomington, IN) and super stiff (Medi-tech, Watertown, MA) guidewires and the Lunderquist exchange wire (Cook, Bloomington, IN). The Lunderquist wire is for nonvascular use only.

Steerable (Torque-Control) Guidewires

Irregular, stenotic, diseased vessels can often be negotiated with a simple-curved angiographic catheter to direct a Bentson guidewire through the diseased segment. When this method is not successful, a variety of new steerable guidewires are available. With these wires, torque applied to the external portion of the wire is transmitted to the distal tip within the vascular system. As a result, with rotation of the wire, the tip can be directed through an area of stenosis. Examples of such wires include the following:

1. Glidewire (Medi-tech, Watertown, MA). The relatively stiff but highly elastic monofilament metallic core of this wire is covered with tungsten-impregnated polyurethane coated with a hydrophilic polymer. This is a very low-friction guidewire when wet. The preformed angled tip can be directed by torque of the external segment. Because of the slipperiness of the wire, a dry gauze pad or specially designed torque device may be required to facilitate guidewire rotation. Its low-friction surface makes the position of this wire less stable than more conventional wires during superselective catheterization.

   A nonvascular use of this wire is negotiation of biliary or ureteral strictures. In general, it should not be used directly through an arterial cannula, since upon retraction of the wire the sharp edge of the cannula can cut into its polymeric coating with the risk of embolization of small particulate debris. The Glidewire is available in a straight or angled-tip configuration in calibers ranging from 0.018 to 0.038 in.
2. TAD wire (Peripheral Systems Group, Mountain View, CA) and Wholey wire (Medi-tech, Watertown, MA). The TAD wire has a 0.035-in. proximal shaft that tapers distally to 0.018 in. and incorporates a platinum tip that is relatively atraumatic and highly visible under fluoroscopy. The straight platinum tip can be manually bent into an angled configuration for negotiation of irregular stenoses.

   The Wholey wire is similar in construction to the TAD wire but has a slightly more flexible platinum tip that may assist in crossing very irregular lesions. The Wholey wire is somewhat more expensive than the TAD wire.

Coronary Guidewires

Small-caliber (0.018 in. or less) monofilament stainless steel wires with flexible platinum tips, initially developed for coronary angioplasty, are utilized with increasing frequency for noncoronary vascular and nonvascular indications. Use of this type of wire with new

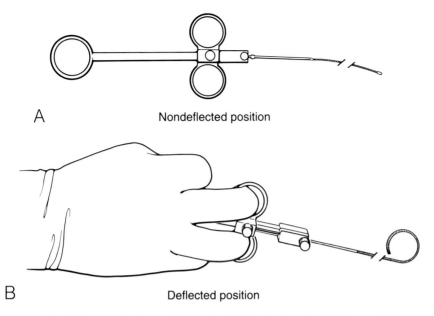

A   Nondeflected position

B   Deflected position

Fig. 4-6. (A) A tip-deflector wire is attached to the deflection handle. In the nondeflected position, the wire tip is straight and somewhat flexible. **(B)** When manual traction is applied to the finger grips of the deflection handle, the tip of the wire forms a closed, somewhat rigid curve of predetermined radius.

coaxial microcatheter (Tracker) systems allows extremely selective positioning of catheters within small, tortuous vessels.

Shorter versions of these guidewires are used in single-stick entry sets for percutaneous biliary and genitourinary procedures.

Lunderquist Ring Wire

This 0.038-in., relatively stiff coil spring guidewire (Cook, Bloomington, IN) is designed for nonvascular use only. The tip can be manually bent to a shape that can be directed by proximal rotation of the wire. This guidewire is most frequently used for biliary and urinary tract intervention. Once the distal flexible end has been completely advanced through a strictured area, its proximal aspect is usually stiff enough to allow for dilator or catheter advancement without buckling.

Tip-Deflector Wire

The tip-deflector wire (Cook, Bloomington, IN) (Fig. 4-6) is designed so that traction on its inner core causes the guidewire tip to bend into a C-shaped configuration. A customized reusable metallic handle attaches to the proximal end of the wire to produce the traction required for tip deflection. With this wire, the radius of the desired tip curvature must be specified (5 or 10 mm). For deflection of catheters within the aorta or inferior vena cava, a 5-mm radius is usually preferable. Because the tip of this wire is relatively rigid when deflected, special care must be taken to avoid vessel trauma during its use.

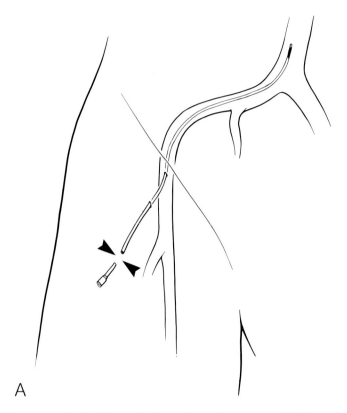

Fig. 4-7. (**A**) The proximal end of the occluded catheter is transected with a scalpel blade to remove the catheter hub. (*Figure continues.*)

Tip-deflector wires are most useful for re-formation of preshaped reversed curve catheters, such as the RH, RLG, and Simmons. Occasionally this guidewire can be an aid in selective catheter positioning. The tip-deflector wire along with a tightly curved catheter may also aid in repositioning central venous catheters and in retrieving intravascular foreign bodies.

GUIDEWIRE INTRODUCTION THROUGH ARTERIAL CANNULAS

Techniques for arterial cannulation were described in the previous section. Once the artery is cannulated, an appropriate guidewire must be introduced to allow subsequent catheter insertion. In adults, a conventional J-tipped coil spring guidewire is generally preferable to reduce the risk of vessel injury. In children, because of smaller vessel caliber and greater propensity for arterial spasm, straight guidewires are used.

VASCULAR DILATORS

Following initial vessel cannulation and guidewire access, coaxial dilation of the subcutaneous tissues and arterial entry site may be necessary to facilitate catheter insertion. Typical vascular dilators consist of thick-walled plastic tubing with tapered tips and a distal luminal

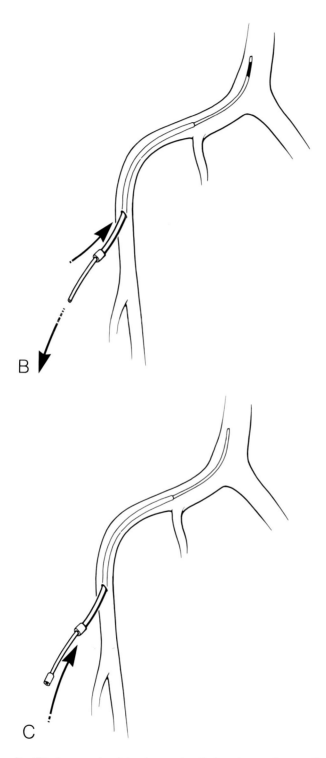

Fig. 4-7 (*Continued*). **(B)** A vascular introducer sheath is advanced over the occluded catheter, which is then retracted through the sheath and removed. **(C)** A new catheter is then introduced through the sheath.

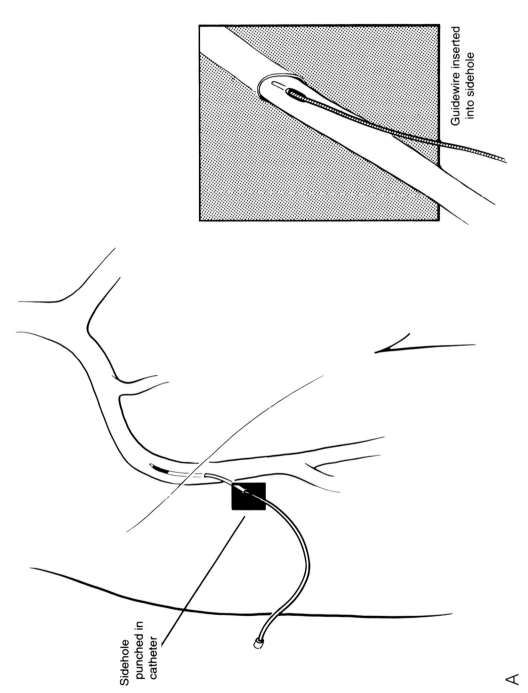

Guidewire inserted
into sidehole

Sidehole
punched in
catheter

A

Fig. 4-8. (A) A guidewire is inserted into a small side hole placed in the catheter wall just outside the skin entry site. (*Figure continues.*)

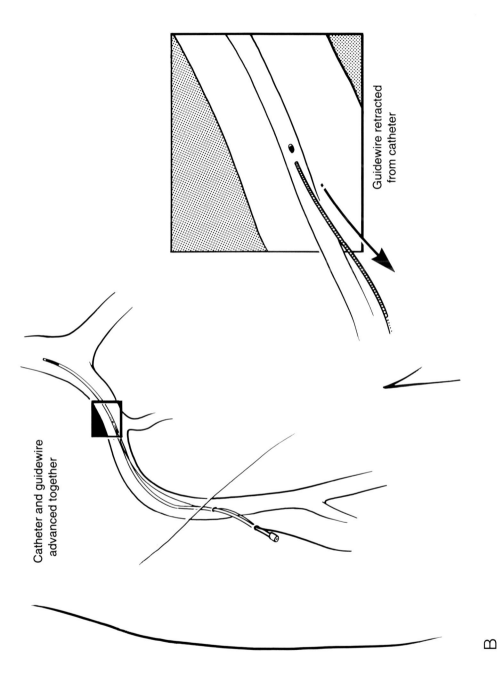

Catheter and guidewire advanced together

Guidewire retracted from catheter

B

Fig. 4-8 (*Continued*). **(B)** The catheter and guidewire are advanced as a unit into the vessel. The guidewire is then retracted slightly to withdraw it from the catheter, which is removed from the vessel. (*Figure continues.*)

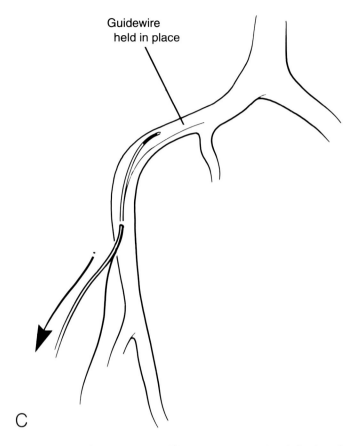

Guidewire
held in place

C

Fig. 4-8 (*Continued*). **(C)** A slightly larger caliber catheter or sheath is then introduced over the guidewire to allow completion of the procedure without any pericatheter bleeding.

orifice closely matching the nominal size of the guidewire over which the dilator is to be used. Vascular dilators are available with proximal Luer lock hubs that allow for flushing and test injections of contrast material. In most cases the nominal outer diameter of the dilator should be equal to or slightly smaller than the nominal outer diameter of the catheter to be introduced. Existence of perivascular scar tissue associated with previous angiographic studies, previous surgery, or the presence of prosthetic graft material may occasionally necessitate overdilation of the arterial entry site by at least one gradation on the French catheter scale.

VASCULAR INTRODUCER SHEATHS

Vascular introducer sheaths consist of two parts: a segment of thin-walled Teflon tubing (the sheath itself) and an accompanying tapered dilator to facilitate introduction of the sheath over a guidewire. Most currently available sheaths have hemostatic membranes to prevent bleeding around catheters or guidewires that have been introduced through the sheath. In addition, a segment of plastic tubing with a three-way stopcock is usually attached as a side arm to the proximal hub of the sheath to allow for flushing, pressure measurements, or contrast injections.

Vascular introducer sheaths may be useful in a number of situations, including the following:

1. Pericatheter bleeding—Exchange of the existing catheter for a sheath with a slightly larger outer diameter will often control the bleeding.
2. Down-sizing an existing catheter—The existing catheter is exchanged over a guidewire for an appropriate sheath. The smaller catheter can then be introduced without pericatheter bleeding.
3. Frequent catheter exchanges—When multiple catheter exchanges are anticipated, patient discomfort and local vessel trauma at the puncture site may be minimized by initial introduction of a sheath.
4. Embolotherapy—When it is anticipated that vaso-occlusive materials (particulate emboli, coil springs) will be injected through a catheter, initial introduction of the catheter through a sheath is generally preferred to facilitate exchange, should the catheter occlude.
5. Replacement of an occluded catheter not initially placed through a sheath—A variety of techniques have been described for exchanging occluded catheters. One such technique involves severing the catheter outside the patient with sufficient length to allow introduction of a relatively tight-fitting sheath over the catheter into the vessel. At this point, the catheter can be retracted through the sheath without loss of vascular access.
6. Catheter introduction through prosthetic graft material.

EXCHANGE OF OCCLUDED CATHETERS

Angiographic catheters may become occluded with blood clot or during intentional introduction of embolic material. When occlusion occurs in a catheter that was not placed through an introducer sheath, special techniques exist for replacing the catheter without sacrificing vascular access. One such technique, described above, is placement of a sheath over the existing catheter (Fig. 4-7). Generally the nominal luminal diameter of the sheath should match the nominal outer diameter of the existing catheter. A relatively tight fit between catheter and sheath must be attained to allow advancement of the sheath through the percutaneous catheter track and vessel wall.

Alternatively, a small side hole is created in the catheter wall just outside the skin entry site to allow the tip of a guidewire to be introduced into the catheter lumen (Fig. 4-8). The catheter and guidewire are then advanced (as a unit) until a sufficient length of guidewire has entered the vessel. At this point the guidewire is retracted slightly to disengage it from the catheter side hole and held stationary at the skin entry site while the catheter is removed. A slightly larger catheter or introducer sheath is then inserted to prevent pericatheter bleeding, and the procedure is completed.

MANIFOLD SYSTEM

For most intravascular procedures, a multiple sideport manifold system (Fig. 4-9) with a port for continuous pressure monitoring, a port providing heparinized saline for catheter flushing, and a port providing contrast for test injections is preferred. A fourth port or a one-way valve in the flush line can be incorporated for attachment to a blood disposal bag to reduce the risk of splash contamination of the angiographer and his assistants during catheter flushing.

A rotating adaptor at the catheter end of the manifold allows rotation of the catheter

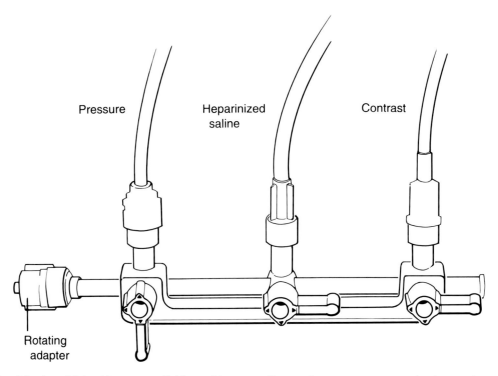

Pressure   Heparinized   Contrast
                saline

Rotating
adapter

Fig. 4-9. A multiple sideport manifold provides a port for continuous pressure monitoring, and ports for flushing and contrast injection during the catheterization procedure.

while it is attached to the manifold. In addition, an assistant can perform test injections of contrast material while the angiographer manipulates the catheter without having to disconnect from the manifold. Between tests, arterial pressure can be continuously monitored and the pressure wave used as an indication of whether or not the catheter tip is free in the vessel lumen. This should prevent forced injection of contrast material through a wedged catheter, reducing the chance of vessel injury.

CATHETER FLUSHING

Intravascular catheters must be flushed with heparinized saline solution frequently enough to prevent luminal thrombus formation that could result in potentially harmful embolic complications. Catheters with multiple side holes, such as pigtail catheters, should generally be flushed more frequently than endhole catheters (every 2 to 3 min). Flush solution should be injected forcefully enough to assure its exit via all the side holes and the end hole of the catheter. When endhole catheters are in selective position, flush solution should never be injected forcefully without first ascertaining that the tip is free within the vessel lumen. This can be confirmed by observing a normal arterial pressure wave form or by free aspiration of blood through the catheter.

Guidewires are relatively thrombogenic compared to catheters. Upon removal of a guidewire from a catheter, a double-flush should be performed by first aspirating and discarding a few cubic centimeters of blood prior to injecting the flush solution.

Nonionic contrast agents disturb coagulation to a lesser degree than do ionic agents. Therefore, the catheter should always be flushed immediately after injection of nonionic contrast material.

REMOVAL OF CATHETERS—SPECIAL CONSIDERATIONS

Pigtail and similar catheters should always be straightened and removed over a guidewire so that the pigtail will not remain coiled in the iliac artery, become compressed, and resist withdrawal through the puncture site. Similarly, reversed curve catheters should be disengaged from selective position by pushing up along the aorta (or vena cava) and then straightened over a guidewire prior to removal to avoid vessel injury caused by advancement of the catheter tip as the shaft is retracted.

If a catheter has been inserted through a prosthetic graft, retraction can cause lengthening and ultimate separation, resulting in a retained intravascular catheter fragment. Removal of the catheter over a guidewire to prevent attenuation of the lumen as it is retracted through the graft wall should effectively prevent separation. As an added precaution, retraction of the catheter should be observed fluoroscopically to ensure that catheter lengthening is not occurring.

SUGGESTED READINGS

Judkins MP, Kidd HJ, Frische LH, Dotter CT: Lumen-following safety J-guide for catheterization of tortuous vessels. Radiology 88:1127, 1967

Kadir S: Diagnostic Angiography. WB Saunders, Philadelphia, 1986

Reuter SR, Redman HC, Cho KJ: Gastrointestinal Angiography. 3rd Ed. WB Saunders, Philadelphia, 1986

Weinshelbaum A, Carson SN: Separation of angiographic catheter during arteriography through vascular graft. AJR 134:583, 1980

5

Complications of Angiography

Kerry M. Link

In addition to reactions related to contrast material, complications related to angiography can be grouped into two categories: those that arise at the puncture site, and those that occur remote from the puncture site. This chapter focuses on complications related to the catheterization procedure itself.

As with all procedures in radiology, knowing the potential complications associated with a particular technique and understanding the mechanism of complications will aid the radiologist in avoiding them, recognizing them when they do occur, and taking steps to rectify, limit, and/or treat their consequences. The complications discussed herein can occur at any puncture site and during catheterization of any vessel. Complications unique to a particular vessel or procedure are discussed separately.

Most angiographic procedures employ the Seldinger method. The entry artery is palpated and then held in position while access is gained via a needle puncture. A catheter is subsequently introduced over an exchange guidewire. Selective catheterization is usually performed with the aid of specialty guidewires. Although these guidewires may be made of different materials with varying stiffnesses and configurations, they can be generally characterized as either straight or J-shaped. This distinction is important, as straight guidewires have a tendency to undermine atherosclerotic plaque and can lead to significant complications. The J-shaped guidewires tend to pass over plaques and should be used in vessels suspected of having or known to have significant atherosclerotic disease.

Catheters are manufactured in a wide array of diameters, shapes, and materials. They may be characterized as having either a single end hole or multiple side holes. With the former, it is extremely important to position the end of the catheter so that it does not rest against a vessel wall. If it does lie against the wall and contrast is injected under pressure, a dissection may ensue. For similar reasons it is important to select a catheter with the proper tip shape and length when selectively catheterizing a particular vessel.

In most instances, the common femoral artery is the entry vessel. Usually the puncture needle passes through both walls of the artery. As the needle is slowly withdrawn, the tip comes to lie within the artery. A guidewire is passed into the artery via the needle, to establish a stable position. The needle is withdrawn, and a catheter is passed over the guidewire into the vessel. It is important to choose a guidewire–catheter combination in which the guidewire is approximately the same diameter as the catheter lumen. A mismatch can lead to difficulty in passing the catheter. Kinking of the catheter as it is advanced over the smaller diameter guidewire, and possible distortion of the catheter tip, can lead to laceration of the vessel at the puncture site, resulting in local hematoma. Similarly, frequent catheter exchanges can lead to vessel laceration; in those cases use of an introducer sheath should decrease the incidence of arterial trauma. In most cases, larger catheter and sheath sizes are associated with an increased incidence of puncture site hematoma or pseudoaneurysm formation, and arterial and catheter thrombosis.

As with all procedures, the longer the time spent in performing the examination, the greater the incidence of complications. This point must always be kept in mind when long studies are planned or when difficulties are encountered during a normal examination.

In all instances, after the examination is completed good hemostasis must be achieved at the puncture site. Failure to do so can lead to a variety of significant local complications that will often require surgical intervention.

ARTERIAL PUNCTURE SITE COMPLICATIONS

Hematoma

In patients undergoing arterial catheterization, 0.25 to 0.50% develop a hematoma that requires surgical intervention. The overall incidence of hematoma is obviously much greater; however, the precise incidence cannot be determined from the records. Since local hematoma is the most common complication associated with percutaneous catheterization, steps must be taken to avoid its occurrence.

Prior to the procedure the patient's prothrombin time, partial thromboplastin time, and platelet count must be evaluated. If the patient is receiving heparin, it should be discontinued prior to the procedure if possible. Similarly, if the patient has hypertension, it must be brought under control prior to the procedure.

Multiple puncture attempts or improper technique can increase the likelihood of local hematoma. A puncture site other than the common femoral artery is associated with an increased risk of hematoma, and large catheters or multiple catheter exchanges also encourage hematoma formation. When multiple catheter exchanges are anticipated, the use of an introducer sheath should be considered.

After the examination, hematoma formation is minimized by manual compression. To be effective, compression must be correctly applied just above the puncture site and for a sufficiently long period of time, usually 10 to 15 min. The use of mechanical pressure devices should be discouraged. Similarly, a pressure dressing can hide oozing blood and is not used routinely.

The nursing staff should monitor the patient closely after the procedure for an appropriate period of time. Frequent visual inspections of the puncture site, as well as hourly monitoring of blood pressure, are necessary. Significant blood loss can occur without the appearance of a hematoma, most commonly as the result of an inadvertent puncture of the external iliac artery, the lateral femoral circumflex vein, or the profunda femoris artery. Puncture of the external iliac artery can lead to significant retroperitoneal hemorrhage and death. Puncture of the lateral femoral circumflex vein or the profunda femoris artery can cause bleeding into intermuscular planes.

Complications of local hemostasis occur more often with transaxillary access since compression is more difficult. Hematomas or pseudoaneurysms requiring surgical intervention occur in approximately 3% of these examinations. The hematoma can compress the brachial plexus and axillary artery, resulting in a compressive neuropathy or axillary artery thrombosis. Therefore, the distal pulses should be checked hourly, along with neurologic examination of the extremity involved. Paresthesia or paresis requires prompt investigation. The incidence of these complications can be reduced by puncturing the distal aspect of the axillary artery, observing strict technique, including a single-wall puncture, with the use of an introducer sheath.

Arteriovenous Fistula

Arteriovenous fistulas develop at the puncture site in approximately 0.01% of patients as a result of simultaneous puncture of an adjacent artery and vein. Even when a single-wall puncture is attempted, the posterior wall of the artery is punctured in more than half of the cases. A fistula develops most often after a high superficial femoral artery puncture that also involves the lateral femoral circumflex vein.

Pseudoaneurysm

Pseudoaneurysms occur in 0.03 to 0.05% of patients undergoing arterial catheterization. They are the result of serious arterial injury that is not controlled with manual compression. Patient characteristics predisposing to pseudoaneurysm formation are similar to those associated with hematoma formation. Predisposing technical considerations include multiple puncture attempts, an inappropriate puncture site, guidewire–catheter mismatch, multiple catheter exchanges, and poor digital compression.

Catheter Thrombosis

Whatever their size, material composition, or type of coating, all catheters are potentially thrombogenic. Platelet/fibrin deposition can be identified on catheters within 15 min after their introduction into the arterial system. Therefore, the longer the procedure, the greater the extent of catheter thrombosis. Once deposition has occurred, it may lead to arterial thrombosis. More commonly, the platelet/fibrin deposit is stripped from the catheter at the puncture site when it is withdrawn. This accumulation may act as a nidus for arterial thrombosis or for distal embolization.

Arterial Thrombosis

Arterial thrombosis is the most common of the serious complications associated with the transfemoral approach. Physical examination indicates that it complicates 0.1% to 0.7% of transfemoral studies, but with Doppler wave or pull-out angiography, the reported incidence is as high as 18%.

Factors predisposing patients to arterial thrombosis include multiple puncture attempts, large-bore catheters, long duration of catheterization, multiple catheter exchanges, and improper compression of the puncture site. The risk increases in pediatric patients because of vasospasm and the large catheter-to-artery ratio. The elderly population is also at risk because of advanced local atherosclerosis and decreased cardiac output. Arterial thrombosis is most often associated with elevation of atheromatous plaques and intimal dissection.

COMPLICATIONS REMOTE FROM THE ARTERIAL PUNCTURE SITE

Dissection

Arterial dissection occurs in 0.64 to 1.75% of studies. Diffuse atherosclerosis is the single most important risk factor leading to dissection. Dissections can occur at the puncture site when the bevel of the needle is not completely within the arterial lumen. When introduced through the needle, the guidewire passes into the subintimal plane. Therefore, it is ex-

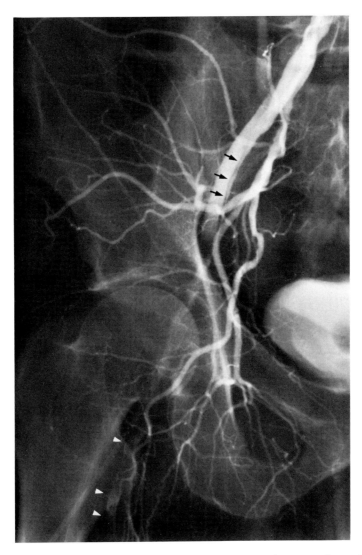

Fig. 5-1. Angiography from a left common femoral artery approach was performed after a patient complained of right leg pain following cardiac catheterization via right common femoral artery entry. An iliac artery dissection (arrows) is present, and occlusion of the common femoral artery has occurred. Thrombus is present in the profunda femoris artery (arrowheads).

tremely important to confirm adequate pulsatile flow through the needle prior to guidewire manipulation. If there is any doubt, gentle hand injection of contrast material can be monitored fluoroscopically to ensure that the needle tip is within the lumen.

Dissection (Fig. 5-1) can occur anywhere distal to the puncture site, even if the guidewire was initially safely introduced into the lumen at the puncture site. Dissection usually occurs as the wire passes beneath an atheromatous plaque and results in a "retrograde" dissection. Therefore, J-shaped guidewires, which tend to "bounce off" atheromatous plaques, are preferred to straight wires, which tend to undermine the plaques. In most cases, this type of dissection will heal spontaneously without surgical intervention. However, dissection in the aorta adjacent to a major vessel can propagate into that vessel or it can occlude its ostium. If a retrograde dissection within the aorta is not recognized and a pressure injection is performed, the dissection can extend proximally and involve several branch vessels with devastating results. Therefore, a test injection should always be performed prior to pressure injection to ensure that a dissection has not occurred, as well as to document catheter position.

Once a retrograde dissection is established, the guidewire may exit the subintimal plane, creating an exit flap cephalad to the entrance site. In these cases, the high pressure within the aorta may undermine the dissection and extend it in an antegrade fashion. The result can be involvement of branch vessels or extension down the iliac/femoral systems.

With an antegrade puncture, any needle or guidewire dissection is in effect an antegrade dissection and can lead to severe problems affecting the vascular tree of the lower extremity.

Arterial Perforation

Arterial perforation remote from the puncture site occurs in 0.1% of studies, usually as a result of guidewire misplacement. Few remote perforations cause significant hemorrhage or pseudoaneurysm formation. However, if a perforation is not recognized and a pressure injection is performed, soft tissue injury secondary to extravascular injection of contrast medium can be significant. Surgical intervention is required when there are cardiovascular symptoms and signs of significant hemorrhage.

Embolization

Embolization is an uncommon complication that occurs in 0.08 to 0.17% of patients. Its incidence increases with the age of the patient. Embolization may result from catheter thrombosis, introduction of foreign material, or disruption of atheroma.

Atheroembolism is the most common mechanism. Advanced age, atherosclerosis, and coronary/aortic arch angiography predispose patients to atheroembolism. Depending on the site of dislodgement, any of the branch vessels can be involved and severe end organ damage may result. Care must be taken not to dislodge atheromata and to flush the catheter on a regular basis.

Translumbar Aortography

Complications follow translumbar aortography in 0.3 to 1.0% of cases. In addition to complications associated with the transfemoral approach, certain rare complications are unique to this technique. Hemothorax, pulmonary infarction, chylothorax, and intrapulmonary hemorrhage may occur when the puncture site is above the T12 level. Paraaortic

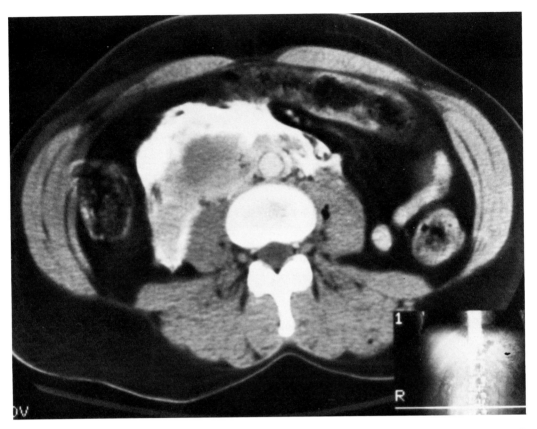

Fig. 5-2. Abdominal computerized tomography was performed in a hypertensive patient who developed severe abdominal pain after attempted translumbar aortography. A large paraaortic collection of contrast material and blood is seen. Symptoms resolved with conservative management.

hematoma occurs in every case, but when patients with hypertension and bleeding diatheses are excluded, hemorrhage is rarely a significant problem (Fig. 5-2). Despite the potential for serious complications, in the absence of hypertension and bleeding disorders, translumbar aortography may be preferable to transaxillary and transbrachial approaches when transfemoral access is not possible.

SUGGESTED READINGS

Hansen KJ, Link KM, Dean RH: Iatrogenic vascular injuries. p. 289. In Bongard FS, Wilson SE, Perry MO (eds): Vascular Injuries in Surgical Practice. Appleton & Lange, East Norwalk, CT, 1991

Hessel SJ: Complications of angiography and other catheter procedures. p. 1041. In Abrams HL (ed): Abrams Angiography: Vascular and Interventional Radiology. Vol. 2. Little, Brown, Boston, 1983

Hessel SJ, Adams DF, Abrams HL: Complications of angiography. Radiology 138:273, 1981

Johnsrude IS, Jackson DC, Dunnick NR: A Practical Approach to Angiography. 2nd Ed. Little, Brown, Boston, 1987

6

Thoracic Aortography

Ray Dyer

Indications: The thoracic aortogram is commonly performed for evaluation of traumatic aortic injury and of dissecting or atherosclerotic aneurysm and for assessment of vessel origins in cerebral or upper extremity vascular disease, including embolism and steal phenomenon.

Risks: Study risks include contrast reaction and site-specific risks of entry. Catheter manipulation in the aortic arch carries a slightly increased risk of stroke. There are rare reports of extension of thoracic tears or dissections with contrast injection.

Catheterization: A 6 Fr 90-cm pigtail catheter is used from the groin, or a 5 Fr 60-cm pigtail catheter is used over a standard J guidewire from an axillary approach. The catheter must be capable of large-volume delivery.

Injection: Contrast material with high iodine concentration is used (350 mg I/ml). A rate of 25 to 35 cc/s for a total volume of 60–80 cc is appropriate. (Routine: 35 cc/s for a total volume of 70 cc.)

Filming Sequence: *Single plane:* 3-4 films/s × 3 s; 1 film/s × 6 s.

Biplane: used for dissection evaluation or with slowed flow. 4 films/s × 4 s; 2 films/s × 4 s. This yields 2 films/s × 4 s then 1 film/s × 4 s in each plane.

Technique: The femoral approach is favored because of the need for a large (6 Fr) catheter. Where dissection or traumatic injury is being evaluated, the pigtail is allowed to form above the iliac bifurcation and advanced into the arch. If obstruction is encountered, a gentle injection should be made to assess position (the false lumen may have been entered, or a complete transection may have been encountered).

If femoral passage appears ill-advised or impossible, an axillary approach is favored. The right axillary route favors entry into the ascending aorta.

The catheter should always be positioned just above the aortic valve so that the valvular sinuses are seen with injection. For dissection, this catheter position aids in determining the type and allows for evaluation of associated valvular insufficiency. This technique demonstrates the coronary arteries because they most often fill from the true lumen. Also, recall that after injury at the aortic isthmus just distal to the left subclavian artery, injury at the aortic root just above the valve is the next most common site.

In the young patient being evaluated for traumatic injury, good cardiac output and tachycardia, often associated with shock, may necessitate a filming rate of 3 to 4 films/s. This rate is difficult to accomplish with biplane filming.

The aortic arch is best evaluated with the patient in a steep 35° to 45° right posterior oblique position. The degree of arch unfolding should be monitored fluoroscopically. The neck and proximal arch vessels should be included on the film, as associated injuries are common.

If further definition is needed, the study can be repeated in a second projection (anteroposterior, left posterior oblique). In these cases, it is better to err on the side of having at least two views.

For dissection evaluation, biplane filming may be adequate. The right posterior oblique position equals the anteroposterior, and the patient is slightly oblique on the biplane lateral. If dissection extends into the descending thoracic/abdominal aorta, consider performing abdominal aortography for definition of the lower extent.

CLASSIFICATION OF THORACIC DISSECTION

DeBakey:
Type I—originates in the ascending aorta and extends into the aortic arch and for a variable distance beyond

Type II—confined to the aortic arch

Type III—originates distal to left subclavian artery origin with variable distal extension

Stanford:
Type A—ascending aorta involved
Type B—arch not involved (distal to left subclavian artery)

SUGGESTED READINGS

Beachley MC, Ranniger K, Roth F-J: Roentgenographic evaluation of dissecting aneurysms of the aorta. AJR 121:617, 1974

Hayashi K, Meaney TF, Zelch JV, Tarar R: Aortographic analysis of aortic dissection. AJR 122:769, 1974

Petasnick JP: Radiologic evaluation of aortic dissection. Radiology 180:297, 1991

Stark P: Traumatic rupture of the thoracic aorta: a review. CRC Crit Rev Diagn Imaging 21:229, 1984

Illustrations

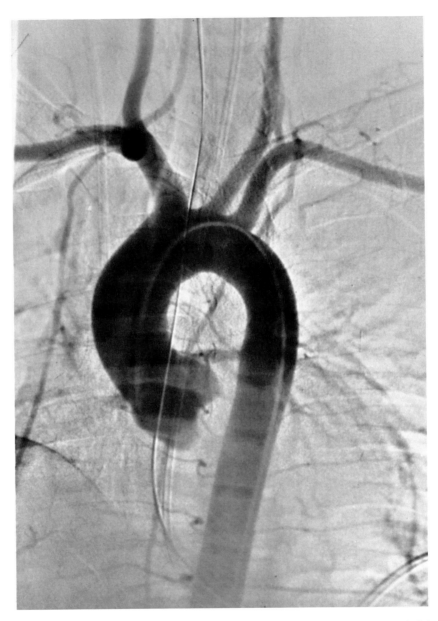

A

Fig. 6-1. (A) Normal thoracic aortogram in right posterior oblique position. **(B)** Labeled drawing of the thoracic aorta. ASA, ascending aorta; AA, aortic arch; DA, descending aorta; BC, brachiocephalic (innominate) artery; LCC, left common carotid artery; LS, left subclavian artery; RS, right subclavian artery; RCC, right common carotid artery; RV, right vertebral artery; LV, left vertebral artery; RIM, right internal mammary artery; LIM, left internal mammary artery; LTC, left thyrocervical trunk; LC, left coronary artery; RC, right coronary artery; I, intercostal arteries.

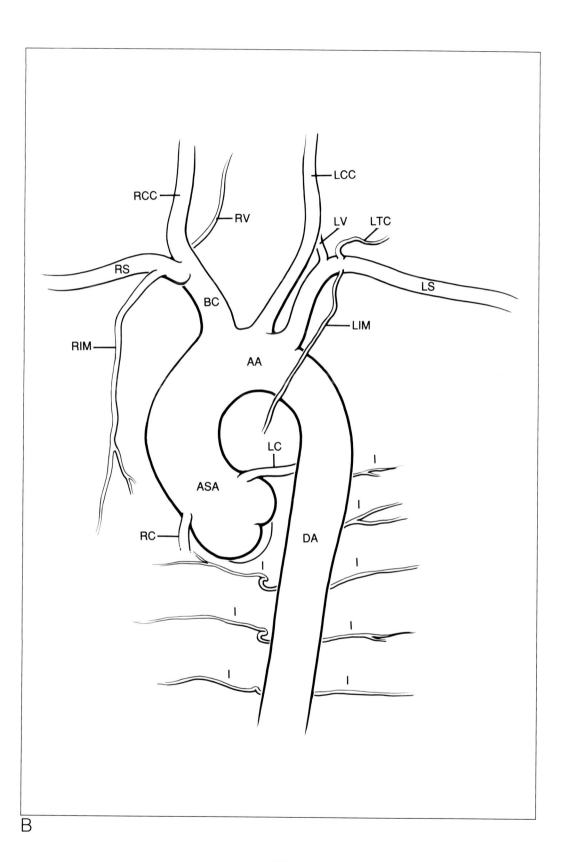

B

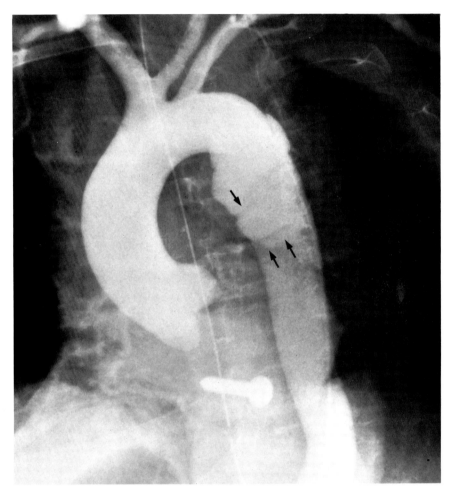

Fig. 6-2. Acute traumatic rupture of the thoracic aorta is present in the classic location. Contour irregularity of the aortic wall is seen, and lucent areas within the contrast column representing intimal tears are also noted (*arrows*).

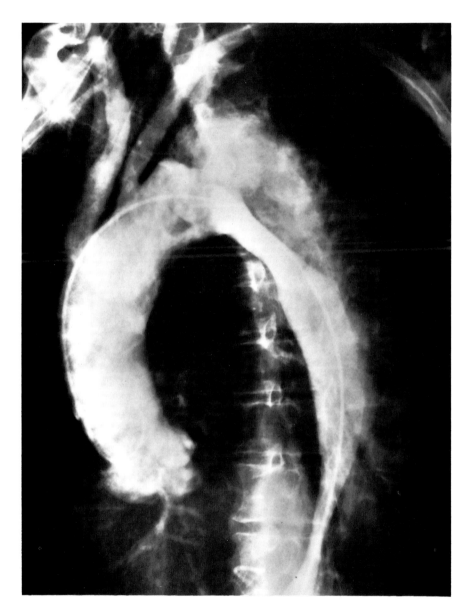

Fig. 6-3. A type III (Stanford Type B) dissecting aortic aneurysm is demonstrated. Note the compression of the opacified aortic lumen by the large intramural hematoma, which begins just distal to the origin of the left subclavian artery.

7

Abdominal Aortography

Ray Dyer

Indications: The usual indications for abdominal aortography are the evaluation of vessel origins in vascular occlusive disease or prior to selective catheterization, and vascular mapping prior to aneurysm repair or other intra-abdominal surgery, such as aorta–extremity revascularization.

Risks: Study risks include contrast reaction and site-specific risks for vascular entry. An upper extremity or translumbar approach may be necessary in patients with lower extremity vascular occlusive disease. Complication risks are slightly higher with this approach.

Catheterization: Catheterization is performed with a 4 to 5 Fr 60-cm pigtail catheter over a standard J guidewire, from the femoral approach. A 90-cm pigtail catheter is necessary for axillary or brachial entry, where a 4 to 5 Fr catheter is favored to reduce complications.

Injection: Contrast material with a high iodine concentration is used (350 mg I/ml). Rates of 15 to 25 cc/s for a total volume of 45 to 80 cc are appropriate. (Routine: 20 cc/s for a total volume of 60 cc). Larger volumes are required for aneurysm evaluation.

Filming Sequence: For routine evaluation, films should be obtained in the anteroposterior plane at a rate of at least 2/s during initial contrast injection. In young patients and patients with tachycardia (>100 beats/min), or when there is specific interest in vessel origins or a suspicion of rapid arteriovenous flow, a filming rate of 3 films/s is necessary. Aneurysmal dilatation will slow vascular flow, and prolongation of the filming sequence will be necessary. Biplane filming technique is useful for evaluating celiac artery, superior mesenteric artery, and inferior mesenteric artery origins and for evaluating abdominal aortic aneurysm. Biplane filming using film changers is limited to 2 films/s in each plane.

Suggested sequence:
Normal flow—single plane:
2 films/s × 3 s; 1 film/s × 4 s; film/2s × 4 s.

Fast flow—single plane:
3 films/s × 3 s; 2 films/s × 1; 1 film/s × 7 s.

Normal flow—biplane:
4 films/s × 3 s; 2 films/s × 2 s; 1 film/s × 5 s (anteroposterior plane only). This yields 2 films/s × 3 s; 1 film/s × 2 s in both planes with five additional anteroposterior plane films.

Aneurysm evaluation—biplane:
2 films/s × 7 s; 1 film/2s × 5 films (anteroposterior plane only). This yields 1 film/s × 7 s in both planes with five additional films every other second in anteroposterior plane only.

Technique: The femoral route is favored because of ease of entry. Aortic disease is often associated with iliac disease. If guidewire passage is obstructed, the guidewire is withdrawn to a stable position below the obstruction and a catheter with a gentle distal curve (JB-1) is introduced. A small amount of contrast material is injected to determine feasibility of negotiation. Alternate guidewires (Bentson, LLT, Glidewire) are then manipulated through the area. The catheter is then advanced, and a small injection of contrast material is used to confirm an intraluminal location and to assess more proximal disease. This method of guidewire advancement–catheter check is used until free passage of the guidewire is obtained. If the catheter occludes an area of tight iliac stenosis during the diagnostic procedure, systemic heparinization is warranted. The neck of an aneurysm may "kink" the abdominal aorta, and it may therefore be necessary to use a catheter to direct the guidewire into the aortic lumen above the aneurysm.

For survey examination, the pigtail catheter is placed above the origin of the celiac artery (T12). Biplane filming is used for evaluation of aneurysm (with a slow filming sequence), aortoiliac revascularization, and vessel origins in mesenteric ischemia or abdominal angina.

Single-plane filming is usually sufficient for survey roadmapping. If the renal artery origins are to be evaluated exclusively, the pigtail catheter should be placed just above the vessel orifices to limit contrast opacification of overlying branches from the celiac and superior mesenteric artery.

If vascular disease precludes femoral entry, a translumbar approach can be used, but this limits possible intervention. The axillary approach is favored if the patient is not markedly obese, has good pulses, and has no coagulopathy. The left subclavian artery provides a less severe transition from aortic arch to abdominal aorta; therefore, a left upper extremity entry is favored.

SUGGESTED READINGS

Chopra PS, Kandarpa K: Arteritides: an angiographic perspective. Appl Radiol 20:13, 1991

LaRoy LL, Cormier PJ, Matalon TAS et al: Imaging of abdominal aortic aneurysms. AJR 152:785, 1989

Muller RF, Figley MM: The arteries of the abdomen, pelvis, and thigh. I. Normal roentgenographic anatomy. II. Collateral circulation in obstructive arterial disease. AJR 77:296, 1957

Rösch J, Keller FS, Porter JM, Baur GM: Value of angiography in the management of abdominal aortic aneurysm. Cardiovasc Intervent Radiol 1:83, 1978

Illustrations

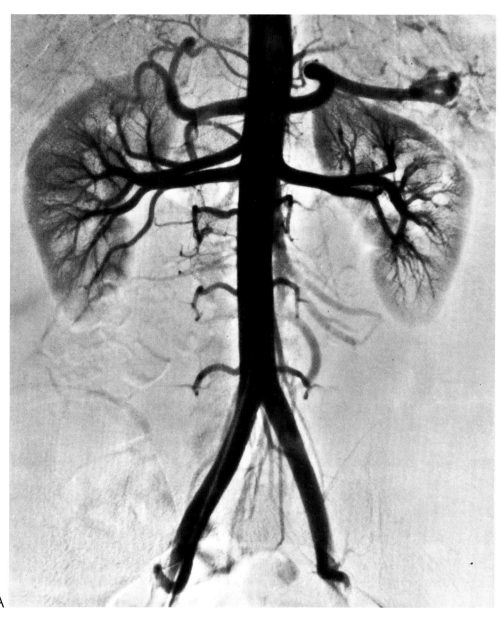

A

Fig. 7-1. (A) Normal anteroposterior abdominal aortogram with two right renal arteries. **(B)** Labeled drawing of the abdominal aorta and branches. *A*, abdominal aorta; *C*, celiac artery; *LG*, left gastric artery; *IP*, inferior phrenic artery; *S*, splenic artery; *CH*, common hepatic artery; *GD*, gastroduodenal artery; *RGE*, right gastroepiploic artery; *PH*, proper hepatic artery; *RH*, right hepatic artery; *LH*, left hepatic artery; *R*, renal arteries; *SM*, superior mesenteric artery; *IM*, inferior mesenteric artery; *L*, lumbar arteries; *CI*, common iliac arteries.

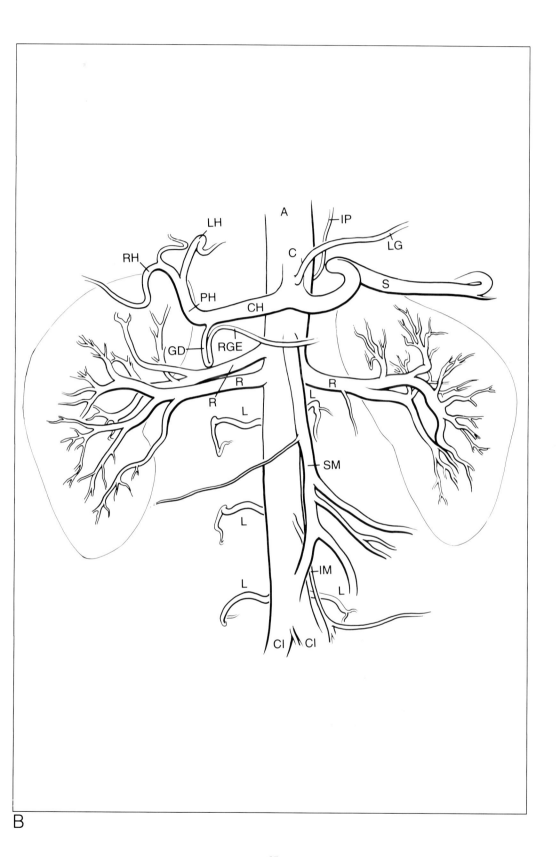

B

65

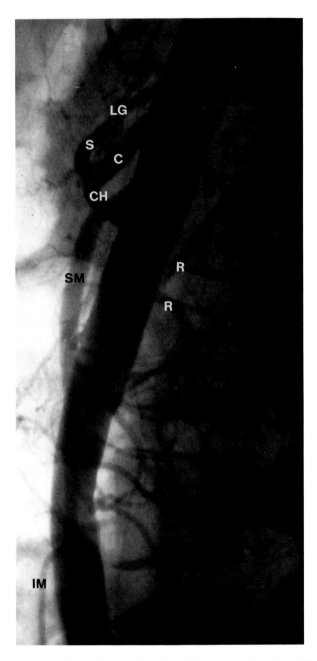

Fig. 7-2. Lateral view of the abdominal aorta showing mild atherosclerotic wall irregularity. *C*, celiac artery; *LG*, left gastric artery; *S*, splenic artery; *CH*, common hepatic artery; *SM*, superior mesenteric artery; *R*, renal arteries; *IM*, inferior mesenteric artery.

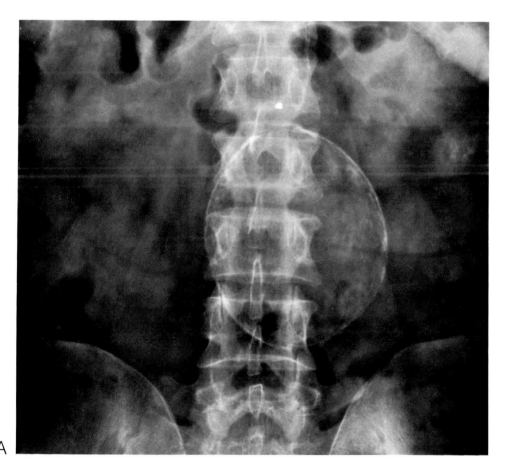

A

Fig. 7-3. (A) An abdominal film in a patient with epigastric pain revealed calcifications in the wall of an 8.5-cm abdominal aortic aneurysm. (*Figure continues.*)

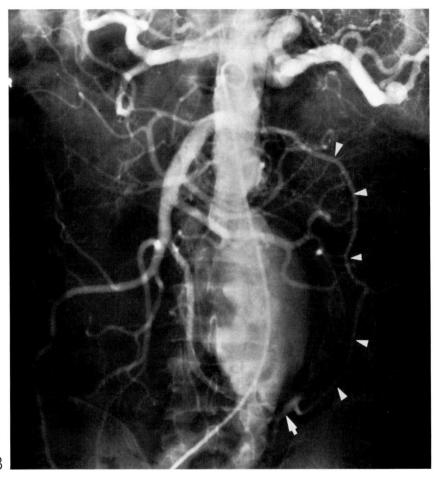

B

Fig. 7-3 (*Continued*). **(B)** Abdominal aortography shows substantial distance between the opacified lumen and calcified aortic wall indicative of mural thrombus. Note the reconstitution of the inferior mesenteric artery (arrow) by a collateral branch from the superior mesenteric artery (arrowheads).

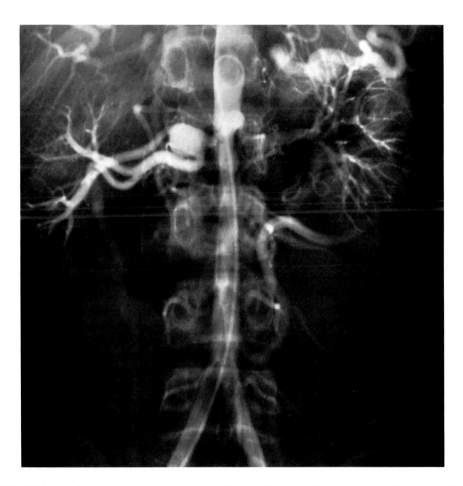

Fig. 7-4. Abdominal aortography in a young patient with acute development of hypertension and elevated erythrocyte sedimentation rate reveals narrowing of both renal artery origins, aneurysmal dilation of the proximal right renal artery, and occlusion of the superior mesenteric artery origin. Diffuse infrarenal aortic narrowing is also noted with an enlarged inferior mesenteric artery supplying collateral flow to the superior mesenteric artery distribution. A diagnosis of Takayasu's arteritis was made.

8

Celiac Arteriography

Mark A. Yap

Indications: Celiac arteriography is performed primarily as a survey examination prior to selective catheterization of a celiac artery branch in the evaluation of visceral tumor, upper gastrointestinal bleeding, or presurgical portal to systemic venous shunting.

Risks: Risks include those associated with arterial access, usually from the femoral route, and intraarterial contrast administration. In addition, there is a risk of dissection or thrombosis of the celiac artery. The clinical consequence is usually insignificant because of the excellent collateral supply from the superior mesenteric artery. However, if the superior mesenteric artery is compromised or if thrombosis extends into the splenic artery, splenic infarction and, rarely, gastric infarction can occur.

Catheterization: Catheterization is performed with a 65-cm RC1 or Cobra 1 or 2 curve, from the femoral route. A 5 to 5.5 Fr catheter is useful if superselective catheterization is planned. If tortuous iliac vessels are present or if a smaller catheter is unstable in the origin of the vessel, a 6.5 Fr RC1 catheter through an appropriately sized vascular introducer sheath may be used.

Injection: A high iodine concentration contrast material is used (350 mg I/ml). The amount and rate of contrast injection are dependent on the size of the vessel, the flow, and any reflux observed during a test injection. Rates of 6 to 10 cc/s for a total volume of 36 to 60 cc are used. (Routine: 6 cc/s for a total volume of 42 cc.) If an endhole catheter is used, a 0.4 to 0.6 s rate rise is employed. If side holes are present, a 0.2 s rate rise is sufficient.

Filming Sequence:	2 films/s × 3 s; 1 film/s × 4 s; 1 film/3 s × 5 films.
Technique:	An anteroposterior projection centered at the midline with the superior margin to include the diaphragm is initially obtained. Variations in anatomy about the celiac axis are common. The catheter is advanced over the wire to the T12 level. The tip is then rotated to an anterior position and the catheter gently retracted until the vessel is engaged. A small amount of contrast material is injected by hand to confirm catheter position. The catheter is advanced slightly to re-form the curve and then tested with a saline injection for stability. Care should be taken to assure that the catheter tip is placed centrally in the lumen to prevent wall dissection during injection.

SUGGESTED READINGS

Baum S, Roy R, Finkelstein AK, Blakemore WS: Clinical application of selective celiac and superior mesenteric arteriography. Radiology 84:279, 1965

Michels NA: Blood Supply and Anatomy of the Upper Abdominal Organs. JB Lippincott, Philadelphia, 1955

Nebesar RA, Kornblith PL, Pollard JJ, Michels NA: Celiac and Superior Mesenteric Arteries. Little, Brown, Boston, 1969

Reuter SR, Redman HC, Cho KJ: Gastrointestinal Angiography. 3rd Ed. WB Saunders, Philadelphia, 1986

Ruzicka FF Jr, Rossi P: Normal vascular anatomy of the abdominal viscera. Radiol Clin North Am 8:3, 1970

Illustrations

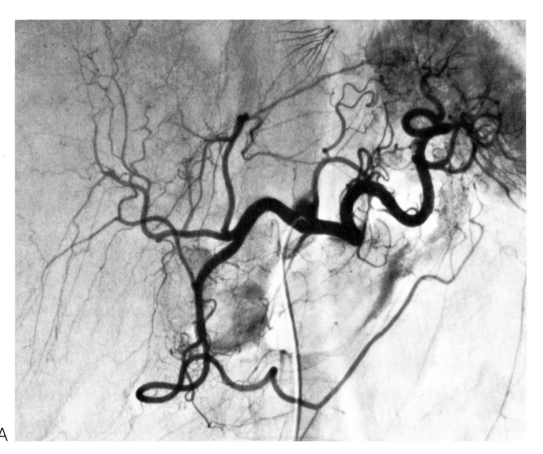

A

Fig. 8-1. (A) Normal celiac arteriogram in the anteroposterior plane. **(B)** Labeled drawing of the celiac artery and branches. *C*, celiac artery; *LG*, left gastric artery; *S*, splenic artery; *SG*, short gastric arteries; *PM*, pancreatica magna artery; *Dors*, dorsal pancreatic artery; *Ubr*, uncinate branch; *Trans*, transverse pancreatic artery; *CH*, common hepatic artery; *PH*, proper hepatic artery; *LH*, left hepatic artery; *RH*, right hepatic artery; *AccH*, accessory hepatic artery; *GD*, gastroduodenal artery; *Post*, posterior superior pancreaticoduodenal artery; *Ant*, anterior superior pancreaticoduodenal artery; *Cys*, cystic artery; *RGE*, right gastroepiploic artery; *Epi*, epiploic artery.

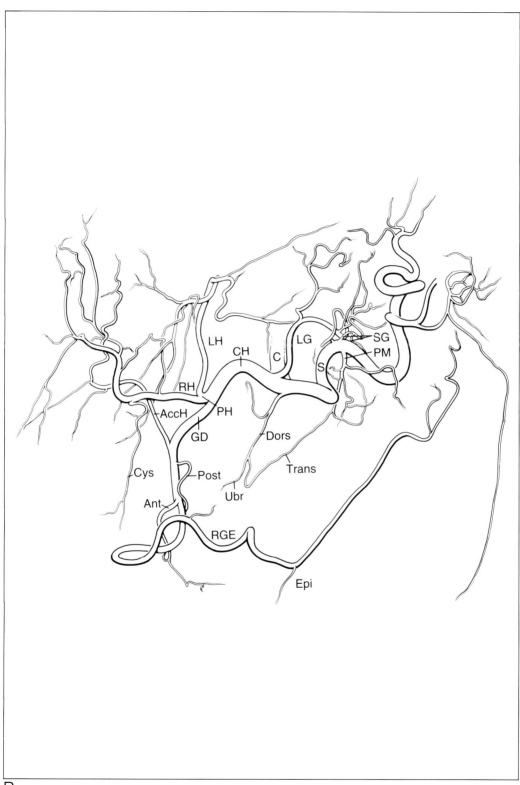

B

9

Hepatic Arteriography

Mark A. Yap

Indications: Presurgical vascular mapping is a common indication for hepatic arteriography. This procedure is performed prior to partial hepatectomy for tumor, prior to placement of a chemotherapy infusion pump, or in preparation for an interventional angiographic procedure such as tumor embolization. Diagnostic evaluation of the hepatic arteries may be performed in the evaluation of portal hypertension, in the differential diagnosis of primary hepatic tumors, and in the evaluation of vascular disease (arteritis, aneurysm), hepatic trauma, or hemobilia.

Risks: Risks include those associated with arterial access, usually from the femoral route, and intraarterial contrast material administration. With selective catheterization of the hepatic artery, dissection or thrombosis may occur. Occlusion of the hepatic artery does not result in hepatic infarction because of the dual blood supply to the liver from the hepatic artery (25%) and portal vein (75%). Duodenal arterial supply also arises from multiple sources (gastroduodenal, splenic, and superior mesenteric artery), so that occlusion of the common hepatic artery does not result in duodenal ischemia unless the other arteries are also compromised. Rarely, hepatic artery occlusion is associated with gallbladder necrosis.

Catheterization: Prior to selective catheterization of the hepatic artery, a survey celiac artery study is performed. The RC or Cobra catheter configuration used for the performance of the celiac arteriogram can usually be advanced over an appropriate guidewire (Bentson, LT, LLT, or Glidewire) that has been placed peripherally into the common or proper hepatic artery. The catheter is advanced over the guidewire using counterclockwise rotation.

Injection: A high iodine concentration contrast material is used (350 mg I/ml). Injection rates in the common hepatic artery of 6 to 8 cc/s for a total volume of 30 to 40 cc are used. In the proper hepatic artery, 4 to 5 cc/s for a total volume of 25 to 30 cc is used. For selective left hepatic artery or gastroduodenal artery injections, rates of 3 to 4 cc/s for total volume of 20 to 25 cc are appropriate. The amount and rate of contrast material injection is highly dependent on the size of the vessel, the flow, and reflux observed during test injection. A 0.4 to 0.6 s rate rise should be used with an endhole catheter. If a catheter with side holes is used, a 0.2 s rate rise is sufficient.

Filming Sequence: 2 films/s × 3 s; 1 film/s × 4 s; 1 film/3 s × 5 films.

Technique: An initial survey celiac arteriogram is performed as outlined in the previous section. For common hepatic artery injection, an anteroposterior filming position is used, centered over the right upper quadrant to include the diaphragm superiorly and the inferior aspect of the liver. Depending on the patient's liver size and body habitus, a 4 to 6 in. magnification technique may be used for better intrahepatic vessel delineation. Oblique views centered over the liver may also be useful when tumors or other processes disturb the anatomic relationships.

All hepatic arteriograms should include superior mesenteric artery injection to evaluate for replaced hepatic (18.5%) or accessory hepatic (6%) arterial supply.

If the RC or Cobra catheter cannot be passed over the guidewire for selective catheterization, a reversed curve configuration such as the Rösch hepatic or Simmons catheter may be useful.

SUGGESTED READINGS

Kadir S: Diagnostic Angiography. WB Saunders, Philadelphia, 1986

Mann JD, Wakim KG, Baggenstoss AH: The vasculature of the human liver: a study by the injection-cast method. Mayo Clin Proc 28:227, 1953

Michels NA: Blood Supply and Anatomy of the Upper Abdominal Organs. JB Lippincott, Philadelphia, 1955

Ruzicka FF Jr, Rossi P: Normal vascular anatomy of the abdominal viscera. Radiol Clin North Am 8:3, 1970

Reuter SR, Redman HC, Cho KJ: Gastrointestinal Angiography. 3rd Ed. WB Saunders, Philadelphia, 1986

Viamonte M Jr, Warren WD, Fomon JJ: Liver panangiography in the assessment of portal hypertension in liver cirrhosis. Radiol Clin North Am 8:147, 1970

Illustrations

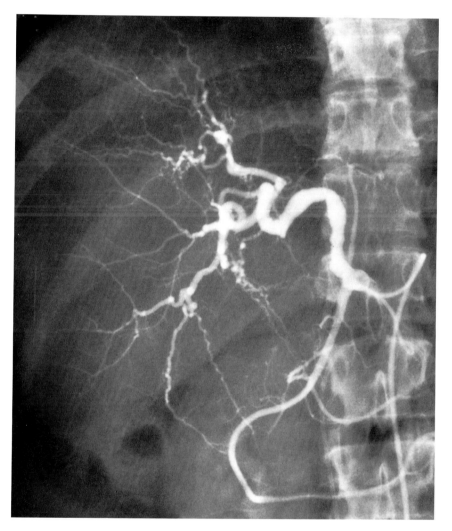

Fig. 9-1. Hepatic arteriography performed during portal hypertension evaluation shows ''corkscrewing'' of hepatic artery branches indicative of fibrotic contraction from cirrhosis.

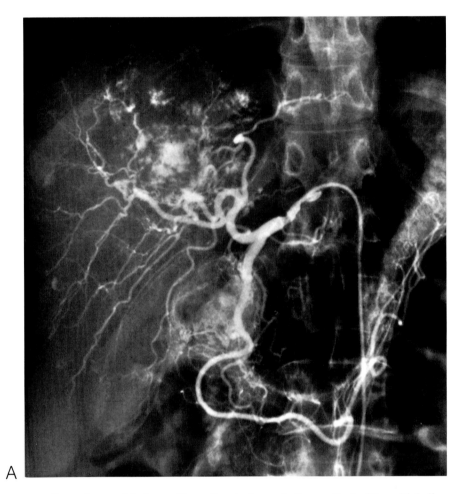

A

Fig. 9-2. (A) The early arterial phase of hepatic arteriography in a patient with multiple liver masses identified at computerized tomography demonstrates multiple vascular "lakes." (*Figure Continues.*)

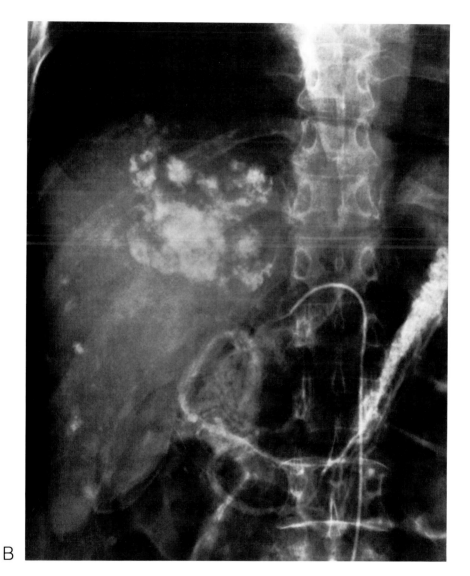

B

Fig. 9-2 (*Continued*). **(B)** Late retention of contrast material in the vascular spaces is typical of hepatic hemangiomas, the most common benign tumor of the liver.

10

Splenic Arteriography

Mark A. Yap

Indications: Splenic arteriography may be performed in evaluation of upper gastrointestinal bleeding or pancreatic processes such as tumor or pseudocyst formation. In addition, assessment of the portal venous system by arterial contrast injection of the splenic artery (in concert with the superior mesenteric artery) and late filming may be performed. Splenic and portal venous opacification can be accomplished by direct contrast material injection into the splenic parenchyma percutaneously, or by transhepatic portal venous catheterization. Arterial portography, which is less invasive, is required for evaluation of mesenteric, splenic, and portal vein patency before surgical shunting; for evaluation of portal hemodynamics (hepatopetal versus hepatofugal blood flow); for identification of gastric, esophageal, or mesenteric varices; or for documentation of shunt patency after surgery.

Risks: Risks include those associated with arterial entry and contrast material administration. Selective catheterization carries a slightly higher risk of vessel dissection or thrombosis.

Catheterization: A 5 Fr RC or Cobra catheter is used. A 6.5 Fr catheter may be necessary to provide sufficient torque control in tortuous vessels and improved stability during injection.

Injection: A high iodine concentration contrast material is used (350 mg I/ml). Injection rates of 6 to 10 cc/s for a total volume of 50 to 70 cc are used (routine: 6 cc/s for a total volume of 54 cc). Higher rates of flow and larger volumes of contrast material are used in patients with splenomegaly. A rate rise of 0.4 to 0.6 s reduces the risk of vessel dissection or catheter displacement during injection.

Filming Sequence:	1 film/s × 10 s; 1 film/2 s × 10 films.
Technique:	The need for a survey celiac arteriogram prior to selective branch catheterization should be considered. It is usually possible to advance the RC or Cobra catheter used in celiac arteriography into the splenic artery over an appropriate guidewire (Bentson, Glidewire, LT). Filming is performed over the left upper quadrant with the diaphragm at the superior extent. A 15° to 20° right posterior oblique position will augment splenoportal venous opacification by gravity. In patients with splenomegaly, higher rates of injection and larger volumes of contrast material should be used. A filling defect in the portal vein (pseudothrombus) may be seen as a result of inflow of unopacified blood from the superior mesenteric vein. Significant hepatofugal flow or portosystemic shunting may reduce opacification.

SUGGESTED READINGS

Abrams HL: Abrams Angiography: Vascular and Interventional Radiology. 3rd Ed. Little, Brown, Boston, 1983

Edwards EA: Functional anatomy of the porta-systemic communications. Arch Intern Med 88:137, 1951

Kadir S: Diagnostic Angiography. WB Saunders, Philadelphia, 1986

Ruzicka FF Jr, Rossi P: Arterial portography: patterns of venous flow. Radiology 92:777, 1969

Illustrations

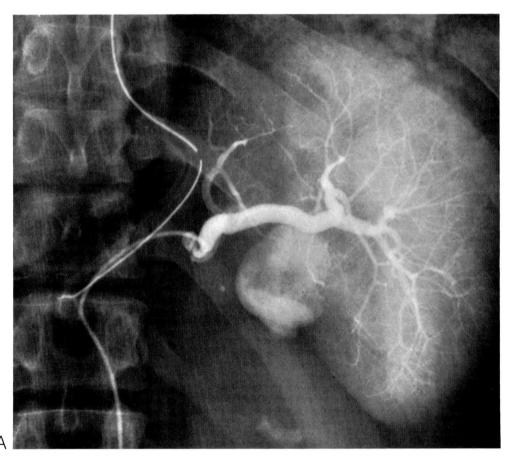

A

Fig. 10-1. (A) Splenic arteriography in a patient with upper gastrointestinal bleeding demonstrates a pseudoaneurysm arising from the midportion of the vessel. (*Figure continues.*)

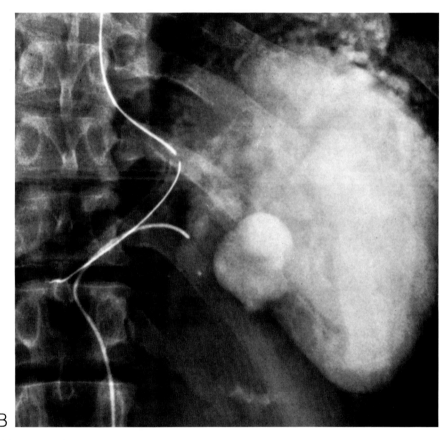

B

Fig. 10-1 (*Continued*). **(B)** Persistence of contrast material in the pseudoaneurysm is seen on the late arteriographic phase. This lesion developed as a result of erosion from a pseudocyst in the pancreatic body.

11

Renal Arteriography

Ray Dyer

Indications:	Indications for renal arteriography include detection of reno-vascular hypertension and differentiation of essential from correctable causes including atherosclerotic stenosis or fibromuscular disease, and arterial thrombosis or embolus, arteritis, arteriovenous fistula, or tumor. Other indications include evaluation of renal trauma, especially with continued bleeding, vascular mapping prior to renal-mass surgery, assistance in diagnosis of the indeterminate renal mass, intravascular therapeutic procedures including percutaneous transluminal angioplasty or therapeutic embolization, evaluation of occult hematuria, and evaluation of potential kidney donors.
Risks:	General risks include those associated with arterial access, usually from the femoral route, and contrast material reaction. Specific risks include branch renal artery spasm, or main renal artery dissection or thrombosis with subsequent renal infarction in selective catheterization. Renal artery rupture during therapeutic procedures has been reported. Selective contrast agent injection into the renal beds is associated with a slightly higher incidence of contrast-induced renal impairment.
Catheterization:	The necessity of abdominal aortography before selective catheterization should be considered. Selective catheterization is performed with a 5 to 6 Fr Cobra, RC, or reversed curve (Simmons) catheter configuration.
Injection:	A high iodine concentration contrast material is used (350 mg I/ml). Rates of 4 to 7 cc/s for a total volume of 10 to 21 cc are

used (routine: 6 cc/s for a total volume of 14 cc). A rate rise of 0.4 to 0.6 s should be used.

Filming Sequence: Blood flow from the renal artery to the renal vein requires 6 to 10 s, and filming should span this time period as a general guide. Where arterial structures are of specific interest, or where fast arterial–venous flow is anticipated, a faster filming rate will be necessary.

Routine:
2 films/s × 4 s; 1 film/s × 4 s; 1 film/2s × 4 films.

Fast flow:
3 films/s × 3 s; 2 films/s × 2 s; then 1 film/s × 7 s.

Technique: Under most circumstances, abdominal aortography should be performed prior to a selective renal artery study. This is essential in evaluation of hypertension, because it is imperative that the origins of the renal vessels be demonstrated. It is important to recall that 25% of patients may have multiple renal arteries, and the entire vascular supply requires delineation for the evaluation of hypertension, neoplasm, and the potential renal transplant donor.

The right renal artery usually takes its aortic origin at the upper margin of the L1 vertebral body, and the left renal artery usually arises slightly lower over the mid-body of L1. The Cobra or RC catheter is advanced into the aorta above the take-off of the vessel, and withdrawn until the vessel of interest is engaged. For intrarenal pathology, multiple views of the kidney are often necessary. Even though the kidney is demonstrated on the anteroposterior aortogram, the small vessel definition is usually insufficient, and it is prudent to repeat the renal arteriogram in the anteroposterior plane initially. Magnification is also helpful for small vessel visualization (4 to 8 in magnification filming, depending on kidney size). A second view, usually obtained in the ipsilateral posterior oblique projection, can be useful in separating the anterior and posterior divisions of the renal artery.

SUGGESTED READINGS

Chait A: Current status of renal angiography. Urol Clin North Am 12:687, 1985
Scott JA, Rabe FE, Becker GJ et al: Angiographic assessment of renal artery pathology: how reliable? AJR 141:1299, 1983
Watson RC, Fleming RJ, Evans JA: Arteriography in the diagnosis of renal carcinoma: review of 100 cases. Radiology 91:888, 1968
Wise KL, McCann RL, Dunnick NR, Paulson DF: Renovascular hypertension. J Urol 140:911, 1988

Illustrations

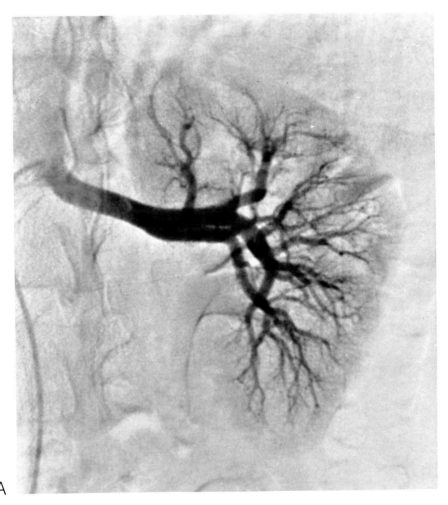

A

Fig. 11-1. (A) Normal selective left renal arteriogram. **(B)** Labeled drawing of the renal artery. LR, left main renal artery; AD, anterior division; PD, posterior division (shaded); AS, Apical segmental artery; US, upper segmental artery; MS, middle segmental arteries; LS, lower segmental artery; PS, posterior segmental artery.

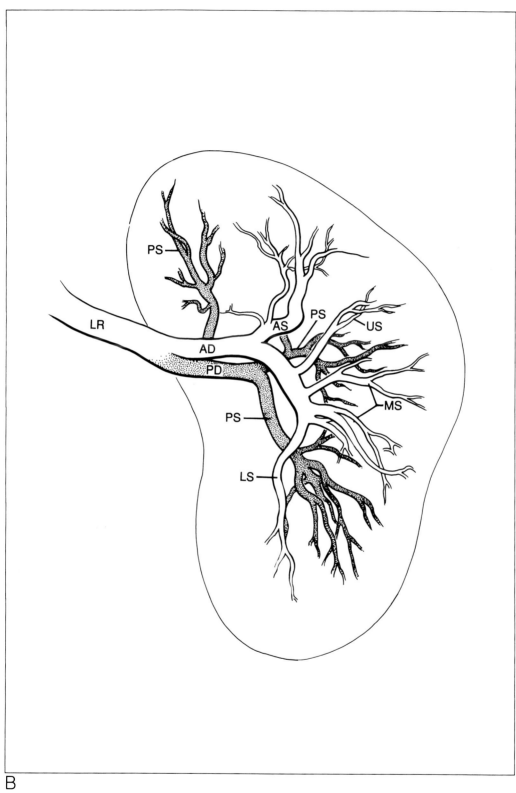

B

93

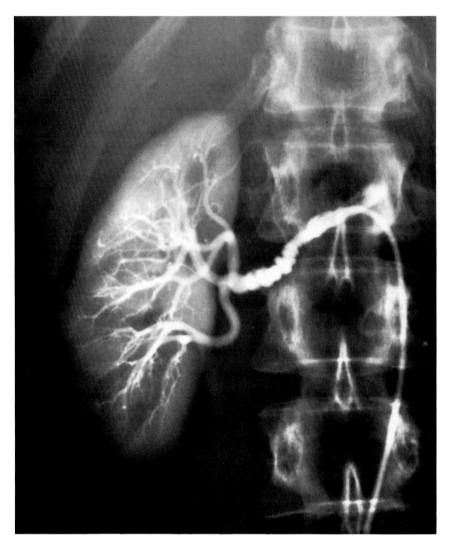

Fig. 11-2. A selective right renal arteriogram in a patient with hypertension shows an irregular contour of the artery described as a "string of beads" appearance from fibromuscular dysplasia of the medial type.

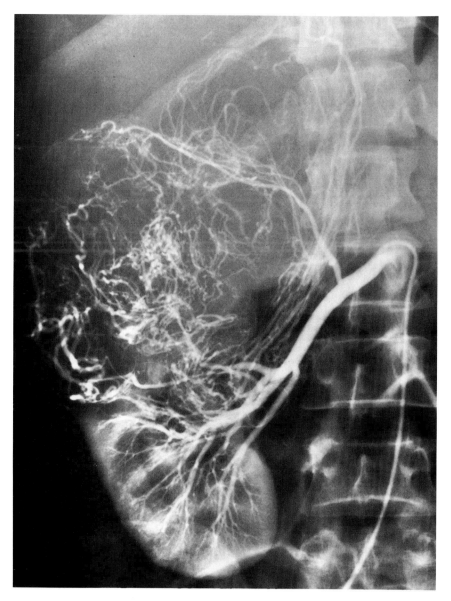

Fig. 11-3. In this patient with hematuria, selective renal arteriography shows gross distortion of the normal arterial branching pattern in the upper pole of the right kidney caused by a large renal cell carcinoma. The linear vessels extending along the course of the right renal vein into the inferior vena cava represent blood supply to intravascular tumor thrombus.

12

Superior Mesenteric Arteriography

Mark A. Yap

Indications: Superior mesenteric arteriography is performed for the evaluation of gastrointestinal bleeding related to diverticula, arteriovenous malformation (angiodysplasia) or tumors, intestinal ischemia from low flow, thrombosis or embolism, or as a part of the workup of portal hypertension to opacify the mesenteric–portal venous structures (arterial portography).

Risks: Risks include those associated with vascular access, usually from the femoral route, and contrast material administration. Selective catheterization carries a slightly higher risk of thrombosis or dissection of the vessel, usually without sequelae because of collateral flow from the celiac and inferior mesenteric vessels. Risks associated with therapeutic intervention such as vasoconstrictor (vasopressin) or vasodilator (papaverine) infusion should also be considered.

Catheterization: Catheterization is performed with a 5 to 6.5 Fr RC, Cobra, or reversed curve (Simmons) catheter.

Injection: A high iodine concentration contrast material is used (350 mg I/ml). Injection rates of 5 to 8 cc/s for a total volume of 36 to 60 cc are used (routine: 7 cc/s for a total volume of 42 cc). Faster rates and larger volumes are used with vasodilator augmentation for the performance of arterial portography (8 cc/s for a total volume 60 cc). A 0.4 to 0.6 s rate rise should be employed.

Filming Sequence: *Standard sequence:*
2 films/s × 3 s; 1 film/s × 4 s; 1 film/2 s × 4 films.

Arterial portography:

1 film/s × 6 s; 1 film/2 s × 12 films. Filming should encompass 20 to 30 s to evaluate superior mesenteric artery–superior mesenteric vein–portal vein flow.

Technique: In patients undergoing evaluation for mesenteric vascular insufficiency or bleeding following surgical aortic reconstruction, biplane aortography for the assessment of vessel origins or aortoenteric fistula should precede selective catheterization. Larger diameter catheters provide improved torque control when tortuous vessels are traversed, or when smaller diameter catheters appear unstable with test injection. Reversed curve configurations are considered the most stable when properly placed, and their use should be considered for prolonged infusion therapy. The Glidewire and Bentson guidewire are useful for superselective catheterization.

Femoral arterial access is established with placement of a standard J guidewire. The catheter is advanced in the aorta to the level of T12 and the tip directed anteriorly just to the left of the midline. The superior mesenteric artery origin is approximately 1 cm caudad to the celiac artery origin. The orifice is usually engaged at the level of the T12–L1 disc space or upper body of L1.

Bleeding at a rate greater than 0.5 cc/min is necessary for angiographic detection of extravasation. A filming sequence is selected to combine rapid early filming and slower late filming to allow detection of the arterial bleeding source and accumulation of extravasated contrast material. Rapid arterial to venous flow may be seen with angiodysplasia.

A slight right posterior oblique patient position (10° to 15°) is used in the performance of arterial portography to project the superior mesenteric and proximal portal vein away from the spine and provide greater opacification of the portal vein due to gravity. Tolazoline, 25 mg diluted in 10 cc of normal saline, is injected via the selective catheter intraarterially over 45 seconds immediately prior to contrast injection. The vasodilatory effect hastens flow from the arterial to venous structures, thereby improving venous definition. Larger doses of contrast material and longer filming sequences are employed.

Intraarterial infusion of a vasoconstrictor (vasopressin) may be used to control gastrointestinal bleeding in appropriate circumstances. After a catheter is placed as selectively as possible into the source vessel, intraarterial infusion with vasopressin is begun at 0.2 unit/min (100 unit/250 cc normal saline yields 0.4 unit/cc). Infusion rates of 30 cc/h (0.2 unit/min) to 60 cc/h (0.4 unit/min) are used. Arteriography is repeated after 20 min, and if bleeding persists, the infusion rate is increased to 0.4 unit/min. Rates in excess of 0.4 unit/min are not warranted. After an optimal rate is established, infusion is continued for 24 h, and the patient is monitored in an intensive care unit setting. If no bleeding occurs, the infusion rate is decreased by half and continued for an additional 12 to 24 h. Vasopressin is then withdrawn and infusion continued with a saline solution for an additional 8 to 12 h. If bleeding recurs at any time during infusion, catheter position should be confirmed.

Infusion of a vasodilator (papaverine) may be used in the therapy of nonocclusive mesenteric ischemia. This condition is generally associated with low vascular flow states and is suggested by the angiographic findings of significant aortic reflux with standard injection rates, slow transit of contrast material to peripheral mesenteric branches, and irregular narrowing of origins or distal branch vessels. Following selective catheterization of the superior mesenteric artery, papaverine infusion is initiated at the rate of 30 to 60 mg/h. Repeat arteriography is performed after 30 min. If mesenteric flow does not appear to be increased or the areas of vasoconstriction improved, the low flow state is considered irreversible. Under these circumstances, surgical exploration should be considered because of the threat of bowel infarction. Some protection may be offered to noninfarcted bowel segments by continuation of the papaverine infusion until the time of surgery.

SUGGESTED READINGS

Athanasoulis CA, Waltman AC, Novelline RA et al: Angiography. Its contribution to the emergency management of gastrointestinal hemorrhage. Radiol Clin North Am 14:265, 1976

Clark RA, Colley DP: Pharmacoangiography. Semin Roentgenol 16:42, 1981

Clark RA, Gallant TE: Acute mesenteric ischemia: angiographic spectrum. AJR 142:555, 1984

Miller KD Jr, Tutton RH, Bell KA, Simon BK: Angiodysplasia of the colon. Radiology 132:309, 1979

Ruzicka FF Jr, Rossi P: Normal vascular anatomy of the abdominal viscera. Radiol Clin North Am 8:3, 1970

Siegelman SS, Sprayregen S, Boley SJ: Angiographic diagnosis of mesenteric arterial vasoconstriction. Radiology 112:533, 1974

Waltman AC: Transcatheter embolization versus vasopressin infusion for the control of arteriocapillary gastrointestinal bleeding. Cardiovasc Intervent Radiol 3:289, 1980

Illustrations

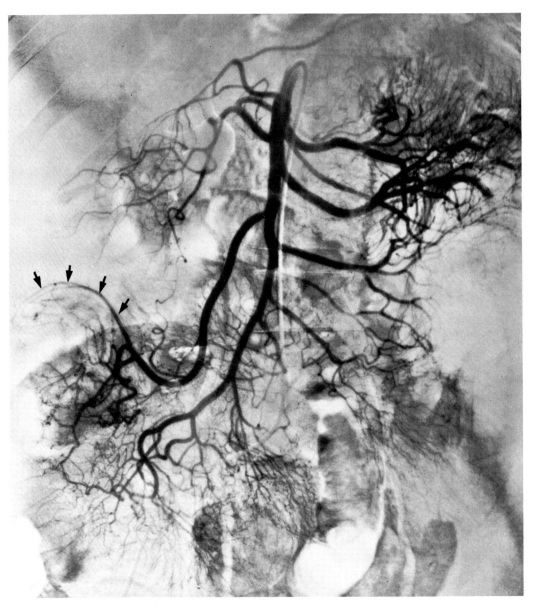

A

Fig. 12-1. (A) Superior mesenteric arteriogram in a patient with a colonic leiomyoma (arrows). **(B)** Labeled drawing of the superior mesenteric artery and branches. *SM*, superior mesenteric artery; *MC*, middle colic artery; *RBr*, right branch of middle colic artery; *RC*, right colic artery; *J*, jejunal arteries; *I*, ileal arteries; *IC*, ileocolic artery; *ABr*, ascending branch of right colic artery.

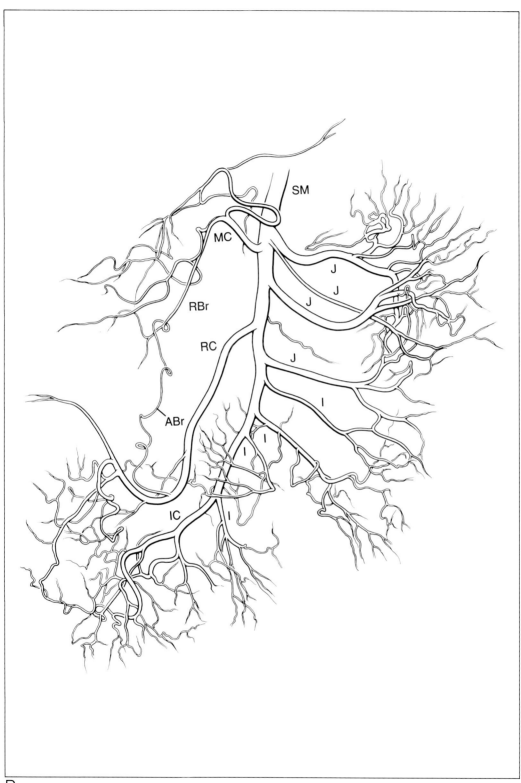

B

101

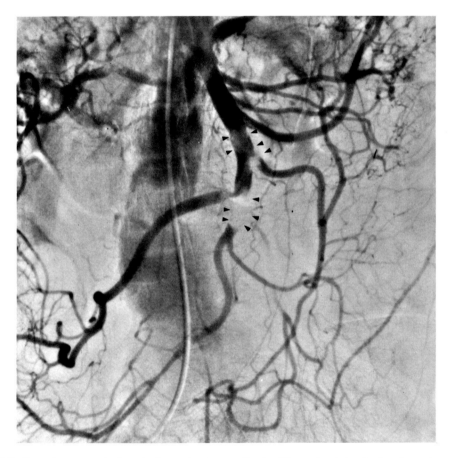

Fig. 12-2. Superior mesenteric arteriography in a patient with acute abdominal pain and previous aortic valve replacement shows multiple emboli (arrowheads).

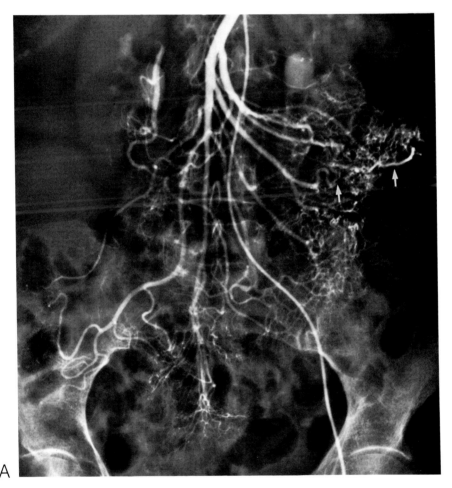

A

Fig. 12-3. (A) The early arterial phase of a superior mesenteric arteriogram demonstrates dilated, tortuous vessels in the proximal jejunum (arrows) in a patient with recurrent gastrointestinal bleeding. (*Figure continues.*)

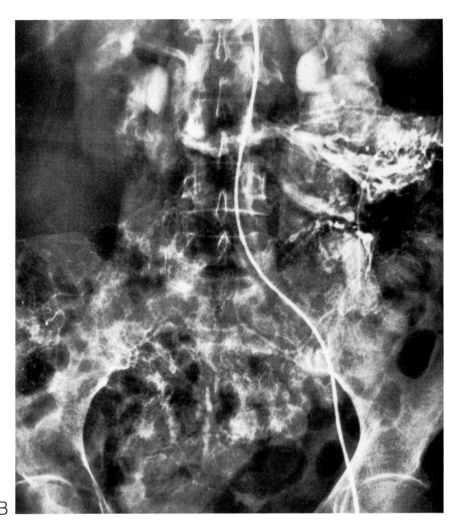

B

Fig. 12-3 (*Continued*). **(B)** Early venous filling is identified from the area of abnormal arterial vascularity, indicative of jejunal angiodysplasia.

13

Inferior Mesenteric Arteriography

Mark A. Yap

Indications: Selective inferior mesenteric arteriography is usually performed for evaluation and therapy of lower gastrointestinal bleeding or ischemia (embolus, arterial/venous thrombosis).

Risks: Risks include those associated with arterial access, usually from the femoral route, and intraarterial contrast material administration. Dissection or thrombosis may also occur with selective catheterization; however, in the majority of individuals, critical colonic ischemia will not occur with adequate collateral supply from the superior mesenteric artery and internal iliac artery branches. Catheter-induced emboli may result in focal colonic ischemia.

Catheterization: A 65-cm 5 to 5.5 Fr RC or Cobra catheter is introduced. If catheterization is unsuccessful using these configurations, a Rösch inferior mesenteric or reversed curve (Simmons) catheter can be employed.

Injection: A high iodine concentration contrast material is used (350 mg I/ml). A rate of 3 to 5 cc/s for a total volume of 9 to 15 cc is injected (routine: 4 cc/s for a total volume of 12 cc). Amount and rate of contrast material injection are highly dependent on the size of the vessel and any aortic reflux observed during the test injection. With an endhole catheter, a 0.4 to 0.6 second rate rise is used.

Filming Sequence: 1 film/s × 7 s; 1 film/2 s × 7 films.

Technique: A standard J guidewire is inserted from the femoral route. The catheter is advanced over the guidewire to the L2 level, and the tip is rotated anteriorly and to the left as it is gently withdrawn. Small test volumes of contrast material are hand-injected to locate the vessel origin, which is usually encountered over the left pedicle of L3. Once the orifice is engaged, the catheter is advanced slightly into the vessel to re-form the curve, and the catheter is tested with a saline injection for stability.

It is often impossible to include the entire inferior mesenteric artery distribution on a single nonmagnified anteroposterior projection. If a bleeding site has been identified by radionuclide scan or endoscopy, this anatomic area should be examined first. If an area of suspicion is not known, the film is centered low enough to include the rectum on the initial injection, and a second injection with filming centered high enough to include the splenic flexure is performed. The distal distribution of the inferior mesenteric artery is examined first to avoid the diagnostic difficulties presented by superimposition of the contrast material-filled bladder. This problem can be remedied to some extent by introduction of a bladder drainage catheter.

SUGGESTED READING

Ruzicka FF Jr, Rossi P: Normal vascular anatomy of the abdominal viscera. Radiol Clin North Am 8:3, 1970

Illustrations

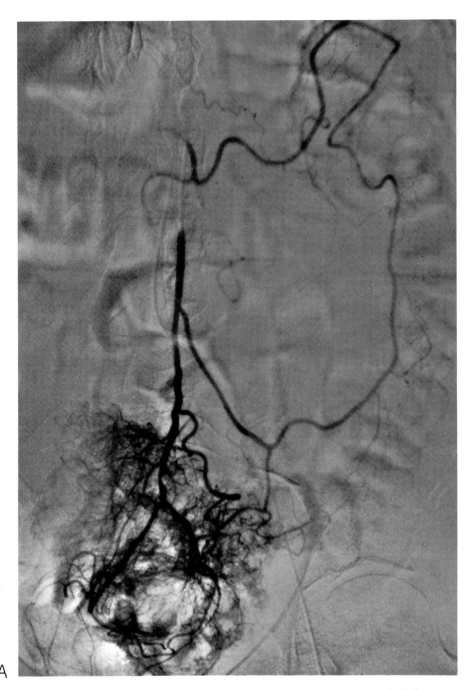

A

Fig. 13-1. (A) Normal inferior mesenteric arteriogram. **(B)** Labeled drawing of the inferior mesenteric artery. *IMA*, inferior mesenteric artery; *LC*, left colic artery; *SH*, superior hemorrhoidal artery; *MC*, middle colic artery (filled retrogradely); *ABr*, ascending branch left colic artery; *DBr*, descending branch left colic artery; *S*, sigmoid arteries.

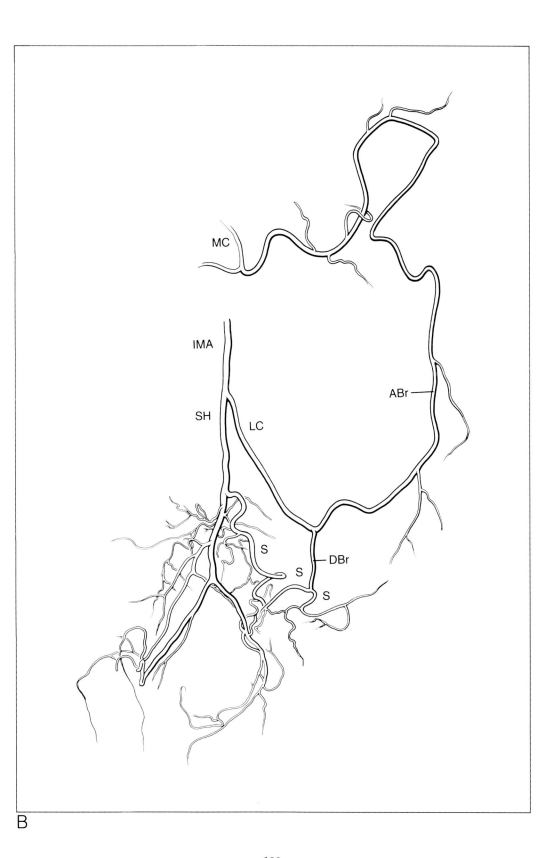

B

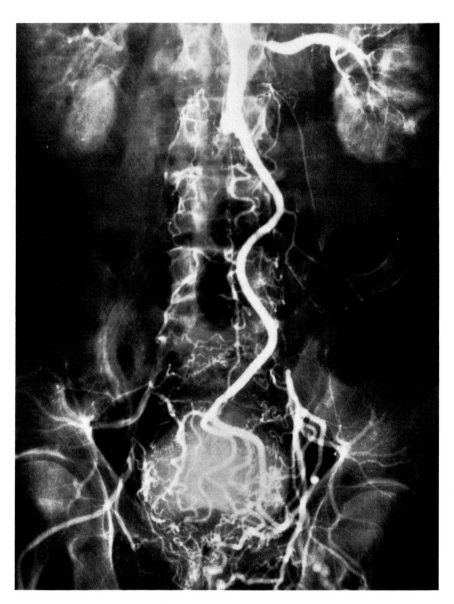

Fig. 13-2. Translumbar aortography demonstrates aortic occlusion. The enlarged inferior mesenteric artery and superior hemorrhoidal branches reconstitute lower extremity vessels via collaterals to the internal iliac arteries.

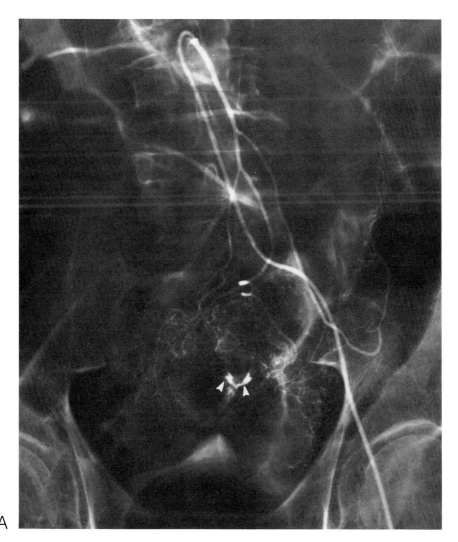

Fig. 13-3. (A) Inferior mesenteric arteriography in a patient with bleeding per rectum shows a site of extravasation (arrowheads) from a superior hemorrhoidal branch. (*Figure continues.*)

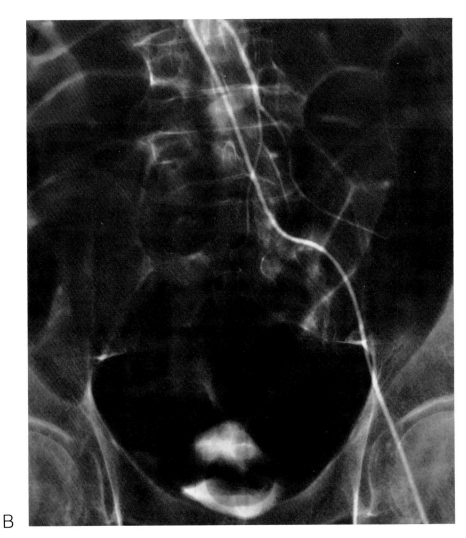

B

Fig. 13-3 (*Continued*). **(B)** Repeat arteriography after infusion of vasopressin at 0.2 units/min for 20 min has controlled the bleeding from a sigmoid diverticulum.

14

Pelvic Arteriography

Ray Dyer

Indications: The pelvic arteriogram may be performed as an extension of abdominal aortography in the evaluation of the extent of aneurysm formation or atherocclusive vascular disease. It is also performed in the evaluation of bleeding from trauma or tumor, vasculogenic impotence, and arteriographic mapping of pelvic tumor or arteriovenous malformation.

Risks: Risks include those associated with vascular entry, most commonly from the femoral approach, and intraarterial contrast administration. Risks associated with necessary therapeutic procedures, such as embolization, should be considered.

Catheterization: A 4 to 5 Fr pigtail catheter is used for the performance of a primary survey study or as a prelude to selective catheterization.

For selective contralateral internal iliac artery entry:
See Chapter 18 for common iliac artery bifurcation crossover technique. A catheter with a gentle primary curve (Cobra or JB-1) is used to select the iliac vessel.

For selective ipsilateral internal iliac artery entry:
A catheter with a tight primary curve (Cobra 2) or reverse-curve (Simmons 2) catheter is used to select the vessel.

A Glidewire is very helpful in selecting internal iliac artery branches.

Injection: A contrast agent with intermediate iodine concentration is used (300 mg I/ml). A nonionic contrast material is suggested for selective arterial injection to reduce patient discomfort.

Survey study from aortic position:
Rates of 12 to 15 cc/s for a total volume of 36 to 45 cc are used (routine: 15 cc/s for a total volume of 45 cc).

Internal iliac artery injection:
Rates of 4 to 6 cc/s for a total volume of 16 to 36 cc are used (routine: 5 cc/s for a total volume of 20 cc). Larger volumes are used in impotence evaluation after pharmacologic augmentation (see below). A rate rise of 0.4 to 0.6 s is appropriate.

Filming Sequence:

Survey pelvic arteriogram with normal flow:
1 film/s × 1 s; 2 films/s × 3 s; 1 film/s × 6 s.

Selective internal iliac artery injection (includes impotence evaluation):
2 films/s × 3 s; 1 film/s × 6 s; 1 film/2 s × 4 films.

Technique:

The femoral route is favored, and the catheter is inserted over a standard J guidewire. For survey examination, a pigtail catheter placed primarily or used in preliminary abdominal aortography is positioned 3 to 4 cm above the aortic bifurcation. Initial films are obtained in the anteroposterior plane. Oblique views are often helpful in evaluating vessel origins, as well as the degree of luminal compromise in eccentric stenosis. A posterior oblique view opens the internal/external iliac artery bifurcation on the ipsilateral side. A contralateral posterior oblique view opens the profunda/superficial femoral bifurcation.

Selective injection into the internal iliac artery is necessary for evaluation of bleeding after pelvic trauma when no source is seen on the survey examination. Selective injections are also required for bleeding or tumor embolization and for evaluation of vasculogenic impotence.

Delineation of the branches of the internal pudendal artery is essential for the evaluation of impotence and can be facilitated by intracavernosal injection of a vasodilator such as papaverine (often in combination with other drugs) or prostaglandin E_1. Filming of the internal pudendal artery and its branches is performed with the patient in a 30° contralateral posterior oblique position and the shaft of the penis taped to the opposite leg. Magnification views may be helpful. Selective internal iliac artery injection is performed as the patient becomes tumescent. Catheterization of the opposite internal iliac artery is then performed, and films are obtained in the other oblique position.

SUGGESTED READINGS

Ben-Menachem Y, Handel SF, Ray RD, Childs TL III: Embolization procedures in trauma: the pelvis. Semin Intervent Radiol 2:158, 1985

Bookstein JJ, Lang EV: Penile magnification pharmacoarteriography: details of intrapenile arterial anatomy. AJR 148:883, 1987

Matalon TSA, Athanasoulis CA, Margolies MN et al: Hemorrhage with pelvic fractures: efficacy of transcatheter embolization. AJR 133:859, 1979

Miller K, Kaplan L, Weitzman AF et al: The radiology of male impotence. Radiographics 2:131, 1982

Muller RF, Figley MM: The arteries of the abdomen, pelvis, and thigh. I. Normal roentgenographic anatomy. II. Collateral circulation in obstructive arterial disease. AJR 77:296, 1957

Illustrations

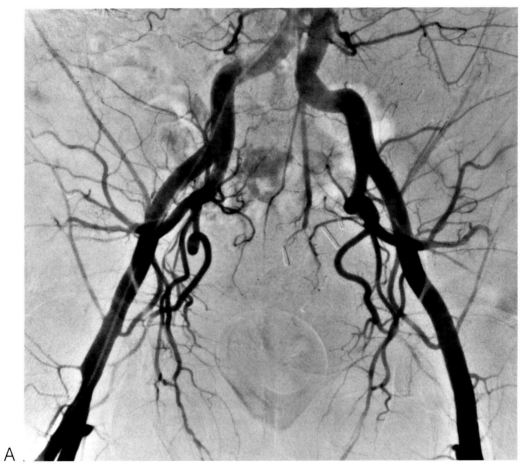

Fig. 14-1. (A) Normal pelvic arteriogram. **(B)** Labeled drawing of the pelvic arteries. *A*, aorta; *CI*, common iliac artery; *L*, lumbar artery; *EI*, external iliac artery; *II*, internal iliac (hypogastric) artery; *DCI*, deep circumflex iliac artery; *IE*, inferior epigastric artery; *SCI*, superficial circumflex iliac artery; *LS*, lateral sacral artery; *SG*, superior gluteal artery; *IL*, iliolumbar artery; *IG*, inferior gluteal artery; *IP*, internal pudendal artery; *O*, obturator artery; *CF*, common femoral artery; *MS*, middle sacral artery; *SH*, superior hemorrhoidal artery (from the inferior mesenteric artery).

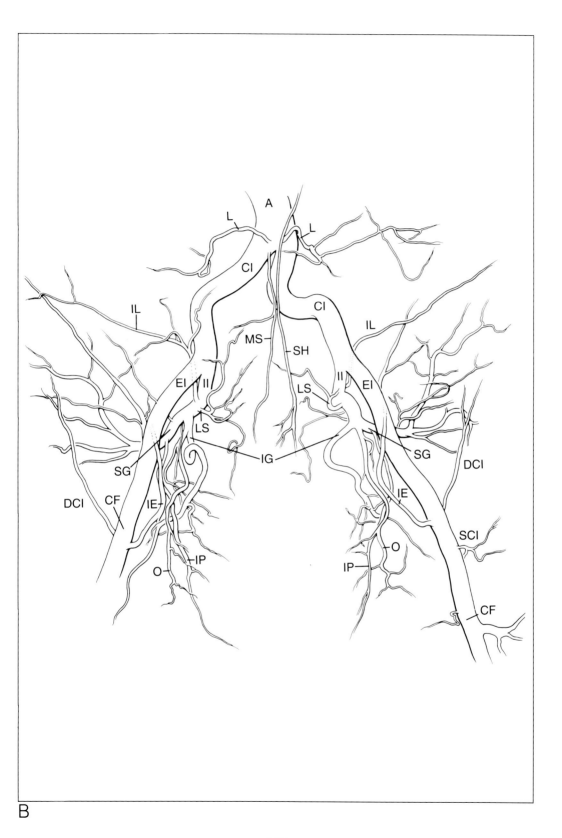

B

117

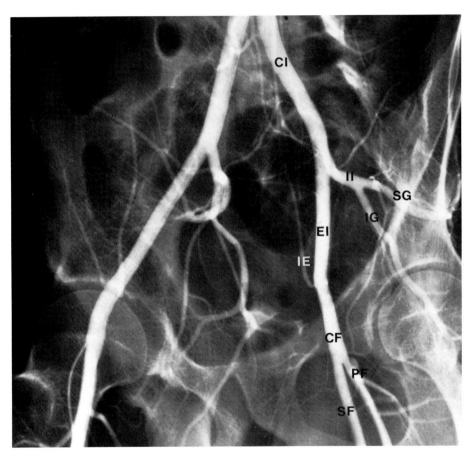

Fig. 14-2. A pelvic arteriogram in the right posterior oblique position shows the right internal iliac and left profunda femoris artery origins to better advantage. *CI*, common iliac artery; *II*, internal iliac artery; *SG*, superior gluteal artery; *IG*, inferior gluteal artery; *EI*, external iliac artery; *IE*, inferior epigastric artery; *CF*, common femoral artery; *SF*, superficial femoral artery; *PF*, profunda femoris (deep femoral) artery.

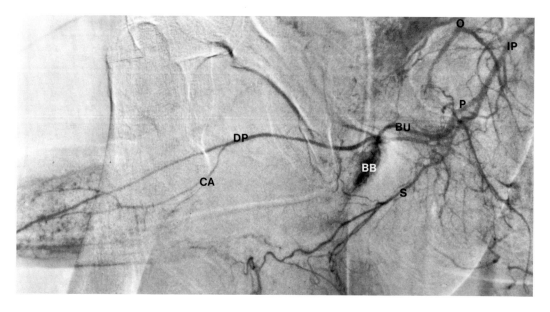

Fig. 14-3. A selective left internal iliac artery injection with filming of the internal pudendal artery and its branches is performed in the evaluation of vasculogenic impotence. *O*, obturator artery; *IP*, internal pudendal artery; *P*, penile artery; *BU*, artery to the bulb; *BB*, bulbar blush; *S*, scrotal artery; *DP*, dorsal penile artery; *CA*, cavernosal artery.

15

Upper Extremity and Hand Arteriography

Mark A. Yap

Indications: Arteriography of the upper extremity may be performed in the evaluation of acute arterial insufficiency (thromboembolism, trauma), chronic arterial insufficiency (subclavian steal, vasospastic disorders), thoracic outlet syndrome, tumor, or aneurysm (see Ch. 16).

Risks: Risks include those associated with arterial access and intraarterial contrast administration. Additionally, cerebral vascular injury may occur as a result of emboli from catheter manipulation or thrombosis. Such injuries are more likely to occur during catheterization of the right subclavian artery as a result of manipulation of the catheter within the innominate artery and the catheter shaft across the origins of the other arch vessels.

Catheterization: A 5 to 5.5 Fr 110-cm Headhunter or Fierstein catheter is used in left subclavian artery studies and in younger patients for studies of the right subclavian artery. In patients with tortuous vessels, a Mani catheter configuration is useful.

Injection: An intermediate iodine concentration nonionic contrast agent (300 mg I/ml) or reduced-osmolality ionic dimer (Hexabrix, ioxaglate meglumine, 320 mg I/ml) is used. Injection rates are dependent on the catheter position.

Subclavian/axillary artery injection:
Rates of 6 to 10 cc/s for a total volume of 18 to 30 cc are used (routine: 8 cc/s for a total volume of 24 cc).

Brachial artery injection:
Rates of 3 to 6 cc/s for a total volume of 12 to 24 cc are used (routine: 5 cc/s for a total volume of 20 cc).
A 0.4 to 0.6 s rate rise is used with an endhole catheter.

Filming Sequence:

Subclavian/axillary artery:
2 films/s × 4 s; 1 film/s × 6 s.

Brachial artery:
1 film/s × 6 s; 1 film/2 s × 6 films.

Technique:

After access is obtained via the femoral artery, the Headhunter catheter is advanced over a standard J guidewire into the ascending aorta. The catheter is rotated until the tip points cephalad and is slowly withdrawn until a vessel origin is engaged. The catheter is advanced over a floppy straight (Bentson) or J guidewire with a 3-mm radius. Distal to the axillary artery, a floppy straight guidewire (Bentson, LLT) and/or vasodilators (nitroglycerin, tolazoline) are employed to reduce vascular spasm. For subclavian and axillary artery injections, initial filming is performed in the anteroposterior projection with the arm close to the side. The proximal brachial artery is included. If a second projection is needed, the tube is tilted caudally at an angle of 15° to 20°.

In thoracic outlet syndrome, anteroposterior projections are obtained with the arm *AD*ducted and *AB*ducted. It is important to decrease the amount of contrast material injected with the arm *AB*ducted, especially if there is evidence of obstruction during a test injection.

Thoracic aortography in the right posterior oblique position with extended filming is performed to evaluate vessel origins in the event of peripheral embolization or the presence of vascular steal.

For evaluation of the brachial artery, the arm is *AB*ducted 60° to 90° and the hand is fully supinated. A second projection can be obtained by pronating the hand and internally rotating the humerus. In cases of suspected trauma, it is useful to do several quick test injections with the arm in different positions to determine the best projection for demonstration of the abnormality. This projection and an orthogonal view are then performed.

HAND ARTERIOGRAPHY

Injection:

An intermediate iodine concentration nonionic contrast agent or ionic dimer is used. Volume and rate of injection depend on the catheter position. For distal axillary or brachial artery injection, 4 to 5 cc/s for a total volume of 20 cc is used. A 0.4 to 0.6 s rate rise is employed with endhole catheters.

Filming: 1 film/s × 15 to 20 s. A filming delay is determined by timing the flow of contrast material from the catheter tip to the area of interest (routine: 2 to 4 s).

Technique: As manifestations of ischemia in the hand may be secondary to a proximal lesion, the arterial supply of the upper extremity from the origin of the subclavian or innominate artery to the forearm should be investigated prior to performance of hand arteriography. For opacification of hand vessels, the catheter must be placed above the brachial artery bifurcation, usually just proximal to the elbow. However, in 14 to 20% of patients, the radial artery and rarely the ulnar artery may arise from the brachial or axillary artery in the upper arm.

Hand arteriography is painful, even with the use of low-osmolar contrast agents. Vasodilators are routinely administered prior to injection to improve vessel delineation. Tolazoline (25 mg) intraarterially 30 s prior to injection may be used. Nitroglycerin (100 μg) may also be used and is often co-administered. Initial films are obtained in the anteroposterior projection with the hand in full supination. A second projection with the hand in partial pronation is useful for distinguishing the origins of the superficial and deep palmar arches.

SUGGESTED READINGS

Calenoff L: Angiography of the hand: guidelines for interpretation. Radiology 102:331, 1972

Coleman SS, Anson BJ: Arterial patterns in the hand based upon a study of 650 specimens. Surg Gynecol Obstet 113:409, 1961

Daseler EH, Anson BJ: Surgical anatomy of the subclavian artery and its branches. Surg Gynecol Obstet 108:149, 1959

Edwards EA: Organization of the small arteries of the hand and digits. Am J Surg 99:837, 1960

Kadir S: Diagnostic Angiography. WB Saunders, Philadelphia, 1986

Illustrations

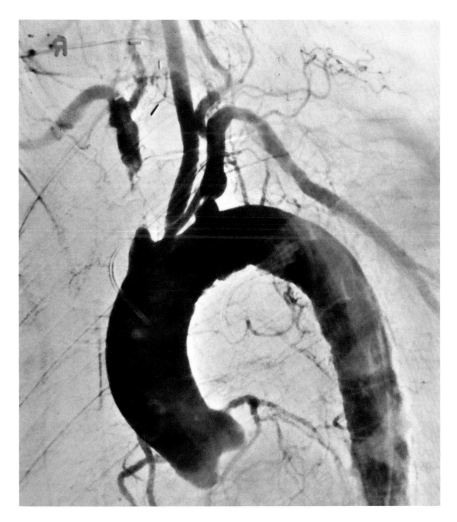

Fig. 15-1. Thoracic aortography performed in a patient who developed left-sided weakness and right arm paresthesias with upper extremity exercise reveals occlusion of the brachiocephalic artery at its origin. Retrograde flow in the right carotid artery fills the right brachiocephalic and subclavian arteries distally (brachiocephalic steal). Note the origin of the left vertebral artery directly from the aortic arch, a normal variant. The right vertebral artery is occluded.

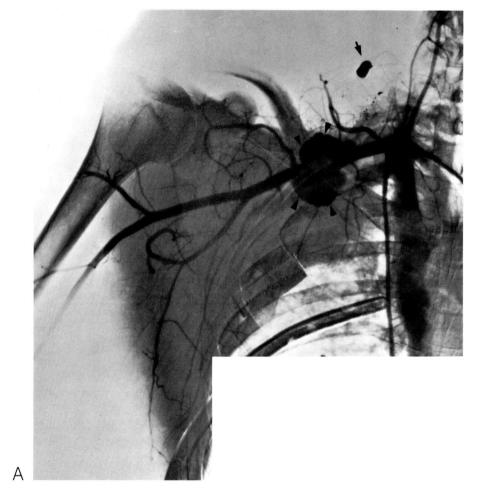

A

Fig. 15-2. (A) Arteriography of the proximal right upper extremity vasculature was performed following gunshot injury to the upper thorax. A pseudoaneurysm is present at the junction of the subclavian and axillary artery (*arrowheads*). A bullet (*arrow*) is seen in the soft tissues of the neck. **(B)** Labeled drawing of the proximal right upper extremity vessels (taken from **Fig. A**). *BC*, brachiocephalic artery; *S*, subclavian artery; *V*, vertebral artery; *AC*, ascending cervical artery; *TCT*, thyrocervical trunk; *IT*, inferior thyroid artery; *IM*, internal mammary artery; *CC*, costocervical trunk; *ST*, superior thoracic artery; *A*, axillary artery; *DS*, dorsal scapular artery; *TA*, thoracoacromial artery; *LT*, lateral thoracic artery; *SS*, subscapular artery; *CS*, circumflex scapular artery; *TD*, thoracodorsal artery; *PHC*, posterior humeral circumflex artery; *AHC*, anterior humeral circumflex artery; *Br*, brachial artery; *PB*, profunda (deep) brachial artery.

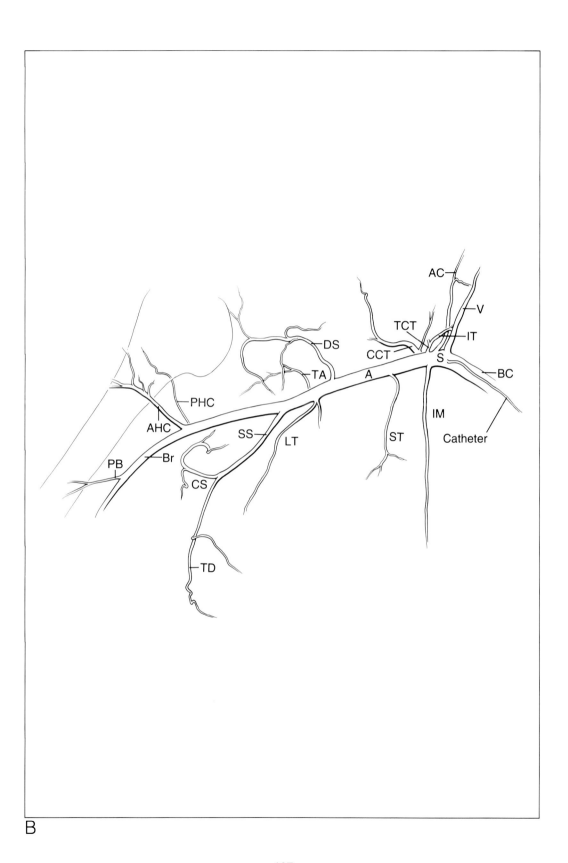

B

127

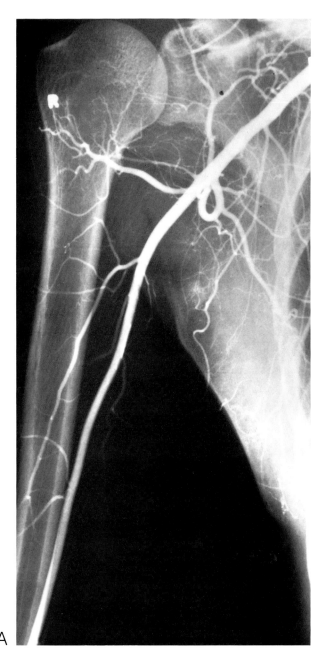

A

Fig. 15-3. (A) Normal arteriogram of the proximal right upper extremity. **(B)** Labeled drawing of the arteries of the upper extremity. *A*, axillary artery; *LT*, lateral thoracic artery; *SS*, subscapular artery; *CS*, circumflex scapular artery; *TD*, thoracodorsal artery; *PHC*, posterior humeral circumflex artery; *AHC*, anterior humeral circumflex artery; *Br*, brachial artery; *PB*, profunda (deep) brachial artery; *SUC*, superior ulnar collateral artery; *RC*, radial collateral artery; *UR*, ulnar recurrent artery; *RR*, radial recurrent artery; *R*, radial artery; *I*, interosseous artery; *U*, ulnar artery.

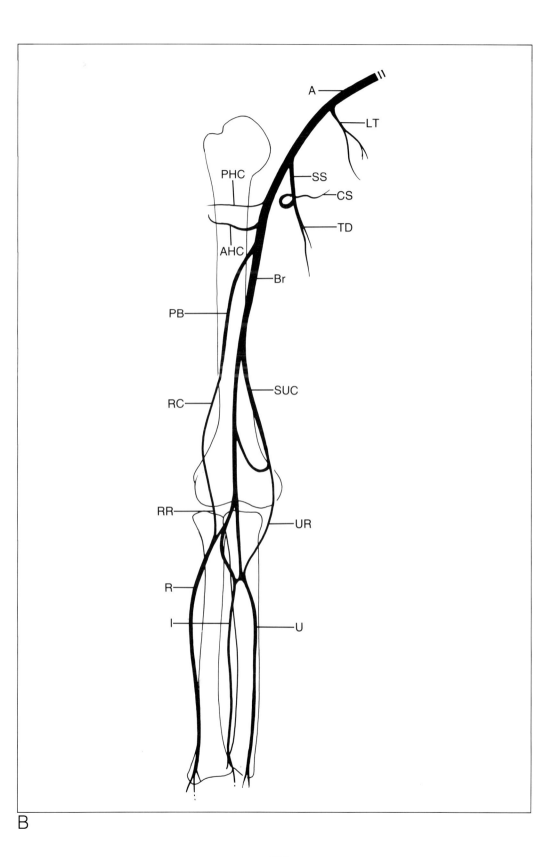

B

129

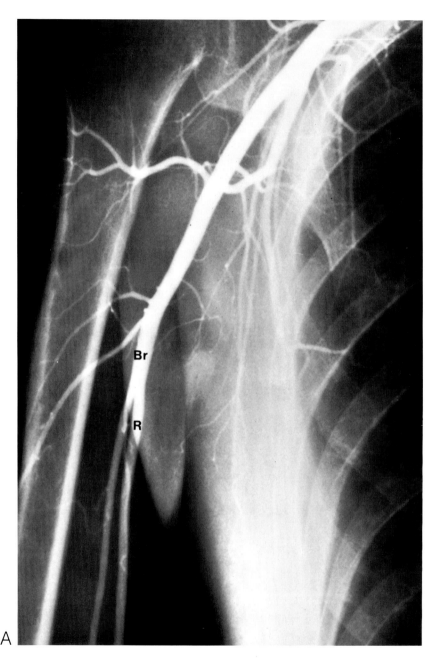

A

Fig. 15-4. (A) Arteriography of the proximal right upper extremity shows a high origin of the radial artery (*R*) from the brachial artery (*Br*). (*Figure continues*).

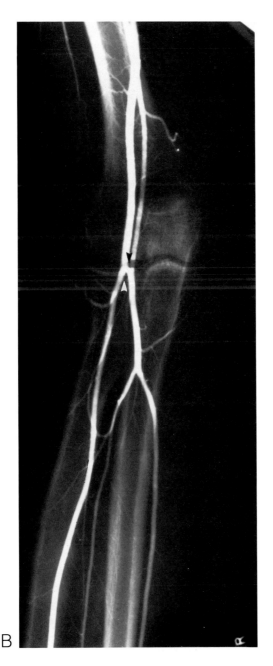

Fig. 15-4. (*Continued*). **(B)** Fusion of the radial (*arrowheads*) and brachial arteries reconstitutes the classic arterial distribution below the elbow.

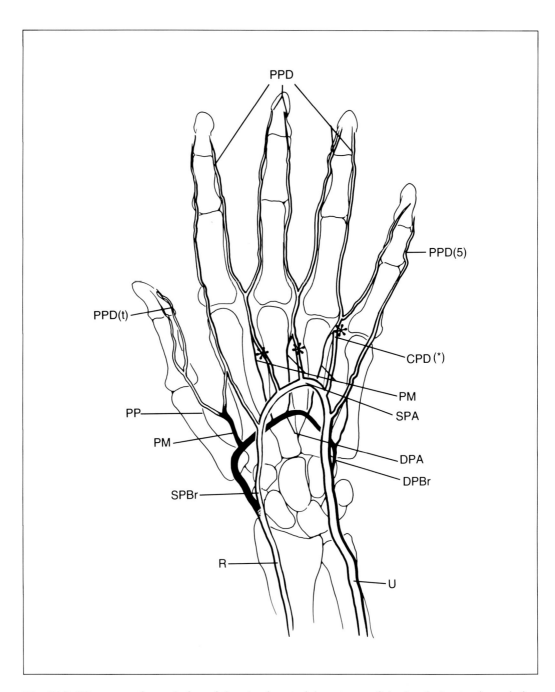

Fig. 15-5. Diagrammatic rendering of the classic arterial anatomy of the hand. Anatomic variation in the hand vasculature is commonplace. *R*, radial artery; *DPA*, deep palmar arch; *PP*, princeps policis artery; *PPD(t)*, proper palmar digital artery (thumb) from deep palmar arch; *U*, ulnar artery; *SPA*, superficial palmar arch; *CPD*, common palmar digital arteries (from superficial arch); *PM*, palmar metacarpal arteries (from deep arch); *PPD*, proper palmar digital arteries; *PPD(5)*, proper palmar digital artery (fifth finger) from superficial arch; *SPBr*, superficial palmar branch (from ulnar artery); *DPBr*, deep palmar branch (from radial artery).

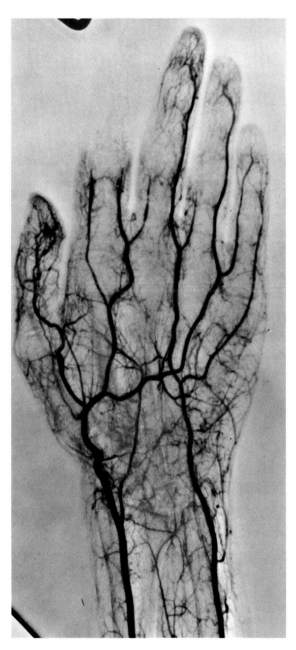

Fig. 15-6. Hand arteriography in a patient with scleroderma and nonhealing finger ulcers reveals occlusions in multiple proper palmar digital arteries despite intraarterial injection of nitroglycerin (100 μg). The superficial palmar arch is incomplete.

16

Dialysis Fistulography

Ray Dyer

Indications: Study of a dialysis fistula is undertaken when difficulty is encountered during dialysis, such as decreased flow, poor venous return, or high venous pressures. Extremity swelling or a change in the palpable fistula thrill may also be an indication for evaluation.

Risks: Puncture of the fistula presents risks similar to other vascular entry sites. The anatomy may dictate a need for catheterization of the inflow artery with site-specific risks. Contrast material reaction is also a risk.

Catheterization: A sheathed needle (Amplatz) or 4 to 5 Fr vessel dilator over an appropriate guidewire can be introduced into the palpable portion of the fistula. Size can be increased as needed for intervention.

Injection: A nonionic contrast agent with intermediate iodine concentration is used (300 mg I/ml). Injection rates of 2 to 6 cc/s for total volume of 15 to 25 cc are used (routine: 5 cc/s for a total volume of 20 cc).

Filming: *Fistula:*
2 films/s × 3 s; 1 film/s × 6 s

Central veins (subclavian—superior vena cava):
1 film/s × 12 s.

Technique: Dialysis fistulas are usually fashioned in the upper extremity. A direct arterial-to-venous communication may be created (most commonly from the radial artery to the cephalic vein), or a graft of synthetic material may be used to fashion the communication.

After 4 to 6 weeks of maturation the fistula can be used for dialysis. The average lifespan of a fistula is 2 years; failure is caused by thrombosis, stenosis of arterial inflow or venous outflow, infection, pseudoaneurysm formation, or distal ischemia related to vascular steal.

The venous side of the fistula is palpated and punctured directly. A blood pressure cuff is placed above the fistula and inflated to 20 mm Hg above systolic pressure. Injection then forces contrast material across the fistula into the arterial side, allowing evaluation. After the rapid filming portion of the sequence, the cuff is deflated so that venous outflow can be filmed.

If it is not possible to place an occluding cuff, or if the fistula is not palpable, it may be necessary to catheterize the source of arterial inflow for evaluation.

The fistula should be studied in two projections. As a rule, the evaluation should include filming over the ipsilateral central veins and superior vena cava to evaluate for associated stenosis.

Interventional procedures such as balloon angioplasty and thrombolysis may significantly prolong the life of these fistulas and one should be prepared to extend the diagnostic evaluation to therapeutic intervention as indicated.

SUGGESTED READINGS

Hunter DW, Castaneda-Zuniga WR, Coleman CC et al: Failing arteriovenous dialysis fistulas: evaluation and treatment. Radiology 152:631, 1984

Hunter DW, So SKS, Castaneda-Zuniga WR et al: Failing or thrombosed Brescia-Cimino arteriovenous dialysis fistulas: angiographic evaluation and percutaneous transluminal angioplasty. Radiology 149:105, 1983

Schwab SJ, Quarles LD, Middleton JP et al: Hemodialysis-associated subclavian vein stenosis. Kidney Int 33:1156, 1988

Tisnado J, Posner MP, Bezirdjian DR: Percutaneous transluminal angioplasty of arteriovenous fistulas in patients on chronic hemodialysis. Semin Intervent Radiol 7:141, 1990

Illustrations

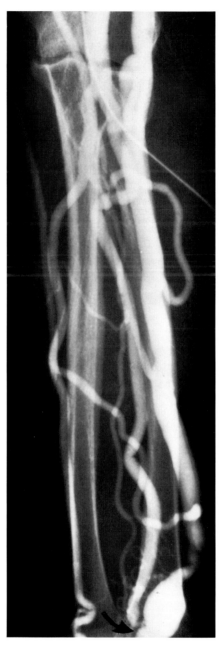

Fig. 16-1. A stenosis (*arrow*) is seen at the anastomosis of a radial artery to cephalic vein (Brescia-Cimino) shunt. Post-stenotic venous dilatation is also identified.

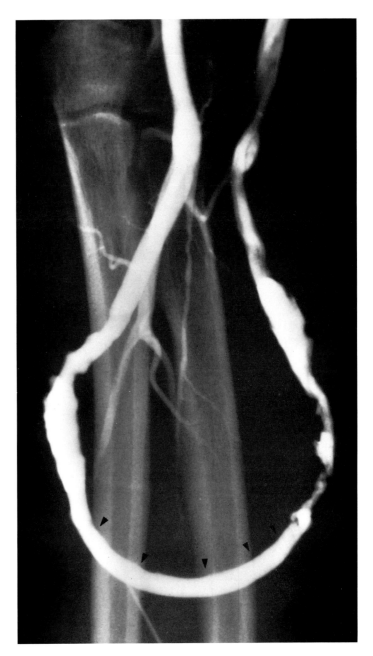

Fig. 16-2. A graft (*arrowheads*) has been inserted between the brachial artery and cephalic vein. Multiple venous stenoses are seen in the native vein as a consequence of repeated puncture.

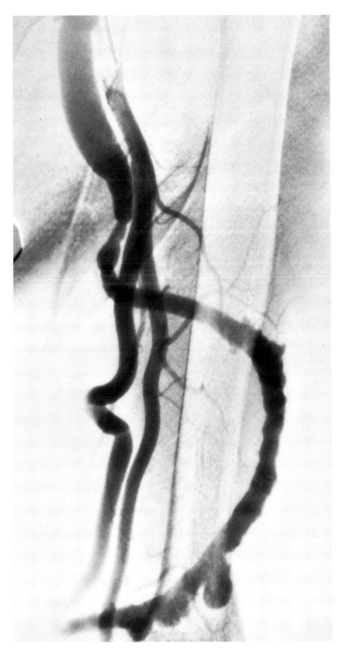

Fig. 16-3. A graft between the radial artery (which has a high takeoff from the brachial artery) and brachial vein shows multiple pseudoaneurysms as a result of repeated access.

17

Bilateral Lower Extremity Angiography

Ray Dyer

Indications: This study is most commonly performed for evaluation and therapeutic planning in chronic or acute arterial insufficiency related to atherosclerotic disease, thrombosis, or embolism. Other indications include evaluation of traumatic vascular injury, arteritis, vascular malformation, aneurysm, or tumor.

Risks: General risks include those related to vascular entry from the femoral, axillary, or translumbar route, and the administration of contrast material. With severe atherocclusive disease, thrombosis or dissection of the common femoral or iliac arteries may occur. A risk of peripheral embolization is associated with negotiation of vessels involved with severe atherosclerotic disease, or with injection of a severely diseased distal aorta.

Catheterization: Catheterization is performed with a 4 to 5 Fr 60-cm pigtail catheter inserted from the femoral route. An axillary or translumbar entry may be required if no femoral access is available.

Injection: An intermediate iodine concentration nonionic contrast material is used (300 mg I/ml). Injection rates should not exceed 8 to 10 cc/s to prevent reflux into visceral branches. The total volume varies from 60 to 100 cc and is dependent on available equipment.

Long leg changer:
The rate is 10 cc/s for total volume of 70 cc.

Stepping table:
The rate is 8 cc/s for total volume of 80 cc.

141

Filming Sequence: Filming sequences are determined by available equipment. In a normal patient, transit of contrast material from the aortic bifurcation to the trifurcation/calf vessels requires 6 to 8 s. In patients with moderate proximal disease, transit time increases to 14 to 16 s. With severe proximal disease and associated distal small-vessel disease, as is often seen in diabetic patients, transit time may increase to 18 to 20 s or longer. Reactive hyperemia generally reduces the transit time and improves vascular delineation.

Long leg changer:
Six films are obtained with an interval of at least 1.5 s between films for film preparation. Because the contrast medium is injected over 6 to 8 s, a filming delay is needed to allow the contrast material to progress distally before the filming sequence begins (2 to 3 s for minimal distal disease, 5 to 6 s for severe disease).

Standard run:
0 s, 3 s, 6 s, 10 s, 16 s, 25 s (Example A, p. 146).

Hyperemic run:
0 s, 2 s, 4 s, 7 s, 11 s, 18 s (Example B, p. 146).

Stepping table:
The filming sequence matches the progression of contrast material down the extremity. An estimate for timing may be obtained by injecting contrast material into the aorta and fluoroscopically monitoring the time required for its appearance at the knee of the leg with less disease. Longer injections give greater latitude in timing and compensate for discrepancies in flow velocity between legs.

Filming sequence: 5 positions/4 shifts (Example C, p. 147).

Pelvis—2 films/s × 2 s
Femur—1 film/s × 3 s
Knee—1 film/s × 3 s
Tibia—1 film/s × 3 s
Ankle—1 film/2s × 4 films

Technique: The femoral route is favored. Access is obtained through the less symptomatic leg with placement of a moveable core or standard J guidewire. Antegrade or retrograde puncture of the more symptomatic leg is then possible if intervention is undertaken. Lower extremity disease is often associated with iliac disease, and the operator should be prepared to negotiate the iliac vessels using techniques described in the section on abdominal aortography. For revascularization planning, or with evidence of distal embolization or proximal aneurysm development, abdominal aortography should be performed in concert with the runoff study.

The tip of the pigtail catheter is placed 3 to 4 cm above the aortic bifurcation to allow equal opacification of the iliac arteries and to prevent reflux into visceral vessels. Proximal iliac occlusion may require opacification of collateral pathways, including intercostal, mesenteric, lumbar, and internal iliac vessels necessitating a different catheter position.

The patient is placed in supine position on the radiographic table with the feet internally rotated. Blood pressure cuffs are placed on the calves, and care is taken to avoid compression of grafts during inflation. The cuffs are inflated to 20 mmHg above systolic blood pressure for 5 to 10 minutes. Upon deflation of the cuffs, reactive hyperemia results. Injection of contrast material should begin immediately after cuff deflation.

Contrast may be "forced" into a side of interest by using hyperemia on this leg, and leaving a cuff inflated proximally on the opposite leg during contrast injection. Arterial vasodilators such as tolazoline or nitroglycerin may be used when cuffs are contraindicated (trauma, grafts). With widely varying flow velocities in the legs, two separate runs may be necessary for adequate delineation.

With the advent of in situ grafting techniques and refinement of interventional vascular techniques, delineation of the vasculature below the knee, including the pedal arches, is necessary for complete diagnostic evaluation and therapeutic planning. The patency of vascular grafts and the success of interventional procedures are dependent in large part on appropriate vessel selection for intervention and patency of distal vessels. Where aortic injection with routine runoff proves inadequate and amputation is contemplated, techniques described in the next chapter should be considered for improved vessel opacification.

SUGGESTED READINGS

Cardella JF, Smith TP, Darcy MD et al: Balloon occlusion femoral angiography prior to in-situ saphenous vein bypass. Cardiovasc Intervent Radiol 10:181, 1987

Darcy MD: Lower-extremity arteriography: current approach and techniques. Radiology 178:615, 1991

Kahn PC, Boyer DN, Moran JM, Callow AD: Reactive hyperemia in lower extremity arteriography: an evaluation. Radiology 90:975, 1968

Smith TP, Cragg AH, Berbaum KS et al: Techniques for lower-limb angiography: a comparative study. Radiology 174:951, 1990

Zagoria RJ, D'Souza VJ, Scharling ES: Prosthetic arterial graft occlusion: a complication of tourniquet use during arteriography. Radiology 167:121, 1988

Illustrations

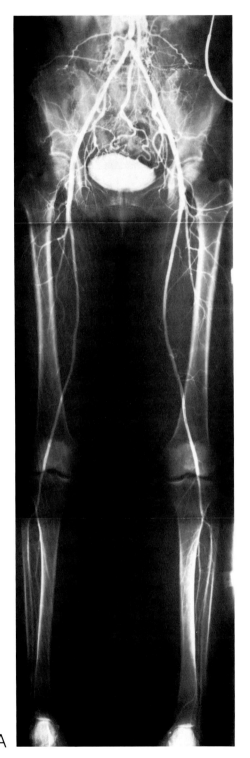

A

Fig. 17-1. (A) Bilateral lower extremity runoff performed with a long leg changer shows near complete occlusion of the aorta proximal to the bifurcation. Enlarged lumbar arteries, inferior mesenteric artery, and its branches provide collateral flow to the lower extremities indicating the hemodynamic significance of the narrowing. **(B)** Labeled drawing of the right lower extremity arteries. *A*, aorta; *CI*, common iliac artery; *II*, internal iliac (hypogastric) artery; *EI*, external iliac artery; *CF*, common femoral artery; *PF*, profunda femoris (deep femoral) artery; *MP*, muscular perforating branches (of *PF*); *LFC*, lateral femoral circumflex artery; *ABr*, ascending branch (of LFC); *DBr*, descending branch (of LFC); *SF*, superficial femoral artery; *DG*, descending genicular artery; *P*, popliteal artery; *LSG*, lateral superior genicular artery; *MSG*, medial superior genicular artery; *LIG*, lateral inferior genicular artery; *MIG*, medial inferior genicular artery; *S*, sural arteries; *AT*, anterior tibial artery; *TPT*, tibioperoneal trunk; *PE*, peroneal artery; *PT*, posterior tibial artery.

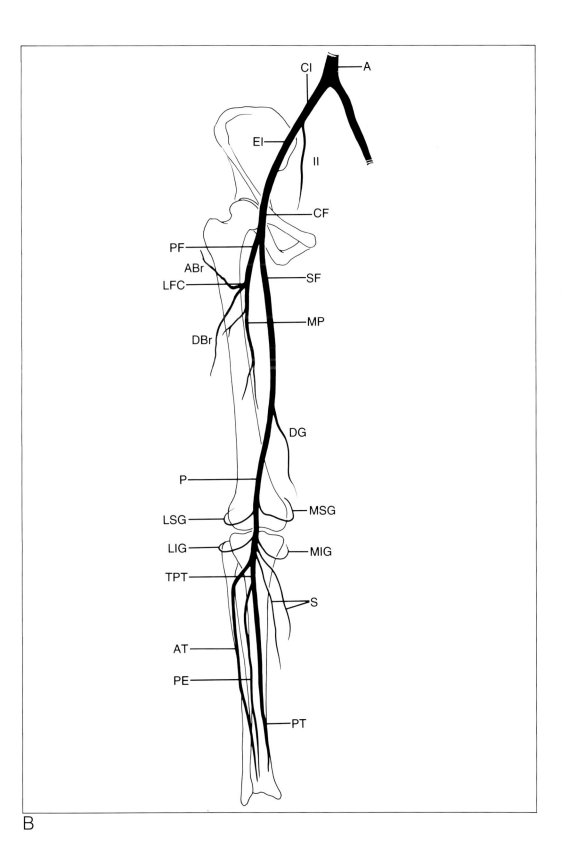

B

145

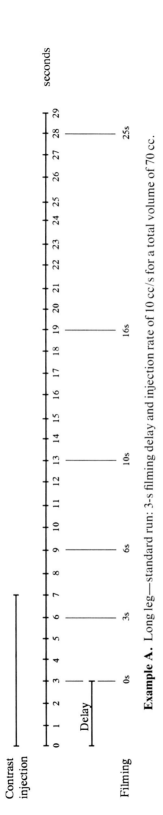

Example A. Long leg—standard run: 3-s filming delay and injection rate of 10 cc/s for a total volume of 70 cc.

Example B. Long leg—hyperemic run: 3-s filming delay and injection rate of 10 cc/s for a total volume of 80 cc.

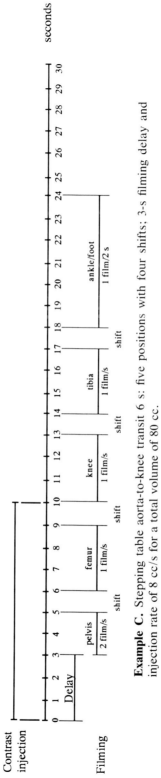

Example C. Stepping table aorta-to-knee transit 6 s: five positions with four shifts; 3-s filming delay and injection rate of 8 cc/s for a total volume of 80 cc.

147

18

Unilateral Lower Extremity Arteriography

Ray Dyer

Indications:

A single leg study is performed for improved definition of vascular structures after a standard runoff procedure, or when interest is confined to one leg, as in the case of traumatic injury, tumor evaluation, embolic occlusion, vascular mapping prior to free vascular flap grafting, or as a prelude to interventional procedures.

Risks:

The risks include those associated with vascular entry and intraarterial contrast administration. As catheter placement proceeds more distally in the leg, risk of catheter-related dissection, thrombosis, or arterial spasm increases.

Catheterization:

Catheter selection is dependent on the site of entry and the indications for the study.

Ipsilateral retrograde femoral entry:
A 4 to 5 Fr straight aortogram catheter with multiple side holes is used.

Antegrade femoral entry:
A 4 to 5 Fr straight endhole catheter or a catheter with gentle primary curve (JB-1) is used.

Contralateral femoral entry:
A 5 to 6 Fr pigtail, RC, Cobra, or reversed curve (Simmons) catheter is used to select the opposite iliac vessel. A guidewire with a long transition (LT or LLT) is directed as far as possible down the iliac artery. The catheter is exchanged over this guidewire. The exchange can be facilitated by ''trapping'' the wire in

the common femoral artery of the leg of interest with manual compression over the groin. Care should be taken to place the catheter tip centrally within the vessel lumen and not against the vessel wall to prevent spasm or vessel dissection during injection.

Balloon occlusion technique with ipsilateral femoral entry:
The procedure is performed with a 6 Fr Berman balloon (Critikon, Tampa, FL) with side holes below the balloon, placed through a 6 Fr introducer sheath.

Balloon occlusion technique with contralateral femoral entry:
A 6 Fr Berman balloon with an end hole is introduced over a 0.032-in. guidewire, placed as outlined above in the description of contralateral femoral entry, through a 6 Fr introducer sheath.

Injection: An intermediate iodine concentration nonionic contrast material (300 mg I/ml) is used. Injection rate will vary with catheterization technique and position.

With the catheter tip in the external iliac artery and approach from either the ipsilateral or the contralateral femoral artery, rates of 5 to 8 cc/s for a total volume of 35 to 60 cc are used. A 0.4 s rate rise is appropriate.

With the catheter tip in the superficial femoral artery from an antegrade femoral approach, rates of 4 to 6 cc/s for a total volume of 20 to 30 cc are used. As the catheter tip is placed more distally in the extremity, flow rates and total volume should be proportionally reduced. A 0.4 to 0.6 s rate rise should be used.

For the balloon occlusion technique with the catheter tip in the external iliac artery and the balloon inflated to stop the flow, rates of 5 to 6 cc/s for a total volume of 30 to 40 cc are used.

Filming Sequence: See Chapter 17 for an outline of long leg and stepping table filming sequences. For a specific area of interest, a rapid film changer can be utilized. For normal flow (after fluoroscopic determination of the radiographic delay, based on transit time of contrast material from catheter tip to area of interest): 2 films/s × 3 s; 1 film/s × 4 s; 1 film/2 s × 4 to 8 films.

Technique: The catheter tip is placed in the external iliac artery of the extremity to be studied after retrograde or contralateral femoral artery entry. This technique minimizes loss of contrast material into the internal iliac artery circulation. Reactive hyperemia can be used to enhance vessel delineation. Long leg or stepping table techniques can be used to survey the vasculature of the entire leg. If a specific area of interest is known, this area can be encompassed with conventional rapid film changers. Two views of vessels in close proximity to traumatic injury should always be obtained for complete evaluation.

Balloon occlusion techniques and high-dose (60 cc) injections in the external iliac artery are useful for improving delineation of small distal vessels, especially in preoperative planning for grafting procedures in ischemic disease. The antegrade femoral approach is most often used as a prelude to interventional radiologic procedures (angioplasty, thrombolysis).

SUGGESTED READINGS

Cardella JF, Smith TP, Darcy MD et al: Balloon occlusion femoral angiography prior to in-situ saphenous vein bypass. Cardiovasc Intervent Radiol 10:181, 1987

Gerlock AJ Jr, Mathis J, Goncharenko V, Maravilla A: Angiography of intimal and intramural arterial injuries. Radiology 129:357, 1978

Smith PL, Lim WN, Ferris EJ, Casali RE: Emergency arteriography in extremity trauma: assessment of indications. AJR 137:803, 1981

Smith TP, Cragg AH, Berbaum KS et al: Techniques for lower-limb angiography: a comparative study. Radiology 174:951, 1990

Illustrations

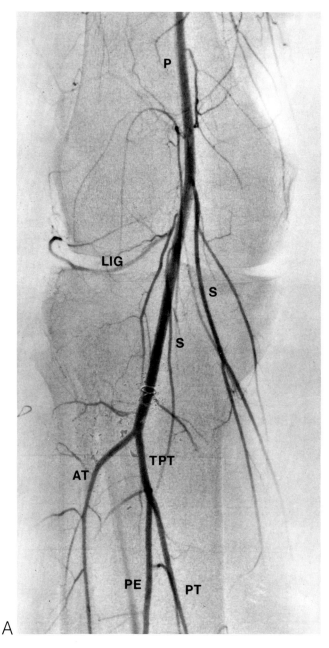

A

Fig. 18-1. (A) Anteroposterior and **(B)** lateral view of the right lower extremity vasculature about the knee was performed after gunshot injury. *P*, popliteal artery; *S*, sural arteries; *LIG*, lateral inferior genicular artery; *AT*, anterior tibial artery; *TPT*, tibioperoneal trunk; *PT*, posterior tibial artery; *PE*, peroneal artery.

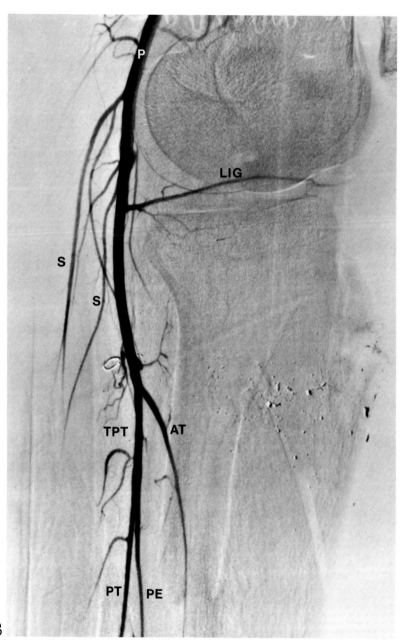

B

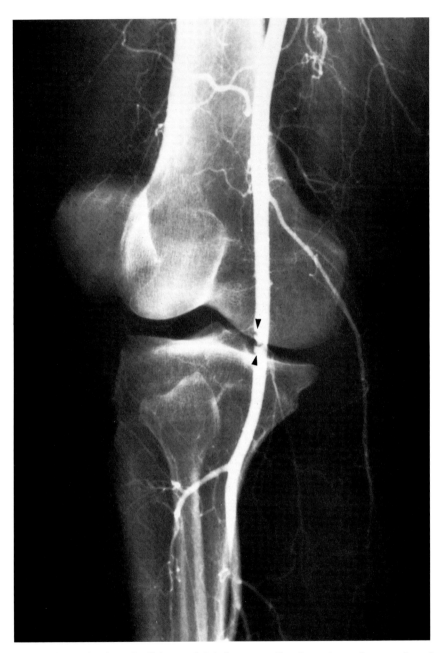

Fig. 18-2. Following reduction of a dislocated right knee, popliteal arteriography reveals an intraluminal filling defect (*arrowheads*) indicative of an intimal tear. Distal pulses were intact.

19

Central Venography and Superior Venacavography

Kerry M. Link

Indications: Central venography of the axillary and subclavian vein is used most commonly in evaluation of venous stenosis or thrombosis, often related to central venous catheterization. The indications for superior venacavography include evaluation of mediastinal disease, including masses and inflammatory conditions, and evaluation of superior vena cava obstruction with development of superior vena cava syndrome from these conditions.

Risks: Risks of the procedure include those associated with venous access and venous contrast material administration. Ventricular arrhythmias induced by catheter manipulation and pulmonary embolism secondary to thrombus or tumor dislodgement during the course of the examination are complications specific to the placement of a central catheter. Detection of venous stenosis or thrombosis may lead to interventional therapy such as fibrinolysis or angioplasty, with the associated risks.

Catheterization: Adequate opacification of the axillary or subclavian vein may be achieved by injection of contrast material through a 19-gauge (or larger) needle placed in a medial vein of the antecubital fossa ipsilateral to the side of interest. For adequate opacification of the superior vena cava, it may be necessary to cannulate both upper extremities to prevent artifacts produced by inflow from nonopacified blood from the noninjected extremity.

If improved opacification is necessary, or if intervention is to be undertaken, a 4 to 5 Fr simple-curve catheter (JB-1) or 4 to 5 Fr pigtail catheter may be placed in close proximity to the area of interest or in the superior vena cava.

Injection: A high iodine concentration contrast material is used (350 mg I/ml). From the antecubital fossa, 10 cc/s for a total volume of 40 cc is injected into the extremity of interest. For opacification of the superior vena cava, similar rates and volumes are injected into each upper extremity.

With a catheter placed in the innominate vein or proximal superior vena cava, 15 cc/s for a total volume of 45 cc is used.

Filming Sequence: *Injection at the antecubital fossa:*
1 film/s × 5 s; 2 films/s × 5 s; 1 film/s × 5 s. The slow initial filming sequence allows contrast material to reach the superior vena cava from the peripheral injection before rapid filming begins.

Central injection:
2 films/s × 10 s. If obstruction is suspected, a filming sequence of 1 film/s × 20 s should be used to demonstrate collateral flow.

Technique: Examination of the axillary or subclavian vein usually begins with cannulation of a vein in the medial aspect of the antecubital fossa on the side of interest. The antecubital fossa is cleansed and draped appropriately. A 19-gauge butterfly needle is placed in a stable position in the vein. Cannulation of veins in both upper extremities may be necessary for adequate opacification of the superior vena cava. From a peripheral location, injection by hand with a 60-cc syringe is preferred to prevent pressure rupture of the butterfly needle.

If improved opacification or other intervention is necessary, the venotomy may be enlarged by passing a 0.025-in. guidewire into the vein through the butterfly needle. The needle is removed, and a small skin incision is made with a #11 scalpel blade. The venotomy is dilated with a 4 to 5 Fr dilator that will accept the 0.025-in. guidewire. Following initial dilatation, a 4 to 5 Fr dilator that will accept a standard 0.035-in. guidewire is advanced into the venous system over the 0.025-in. guidewire. The 0.025-in. guidewire is then removed, and a 0.035-in. guidewire inserted. An appropriate catheter is then placed for completion of the study. A 4 to 5 Fr pigtail catheter can be placed for improved opacification, or a JB-1 catheter can be manipulated into the clot or through a stenotic lesion, if necessary.

Anteroposterior and lateral projections of the superior mediastinum to include both pulmonary hilar areas should be obtained to evaluate for superior vena caval obstruction or compression caused by mediastinal masses. If superior vena caval obstruction is under evaluation, filming sequences should be lengthened to at least 15 to 20 s to provide full demonstration of collateral flow.

Cannulation of a vein of the medial aspect of the antecubital fossa is favored. Entry into the cephalic vein on the lateral portion of the antecubital fossa may complicate manipulation of a catheter into the superior vena cava from the arm, owing to the acute angulation of the cephalic vein entry into the axillary vein.

SUGGESTED READINGS

Gomes MN, Hufnagel CA: Superior vena cava obstruction: a review of the literature and report of 2 cases due to benign intrathoracic tumors. Ann Thorac Surg 20:344, 1975

Lochridge SK, Knibbe WP, Doty DB: Obstruction of the superior vena cava. Surgery 85:14, 1979

Mitchell SE, Clark RA: Complications of central venous catheterization. AJR 133:467, 1979

Rosenberger A, Adler O: Superior vena cava syndrome: a new radiologic approach to diagnosis. Cardiovasc Intervent Radiol 3:127, 1980

Webb WR, Gamsu G, Rohlfing BM: Catheter venography in the superior vena cava syndrome. AJR 129:146, 1977

Illustrations

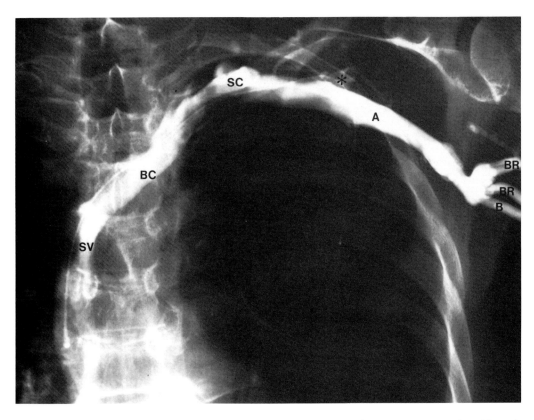

Fig. 19-1. Central venogram from the left upper extremity. *SV*, superior vena cava; *BC*, brachioceph-alic (innominate) vein; *SC*, subclavian vein; *A*, axillary vein; *B*, basilic vein; *BR*, brachial veins; *, inflow from cephalic vein.

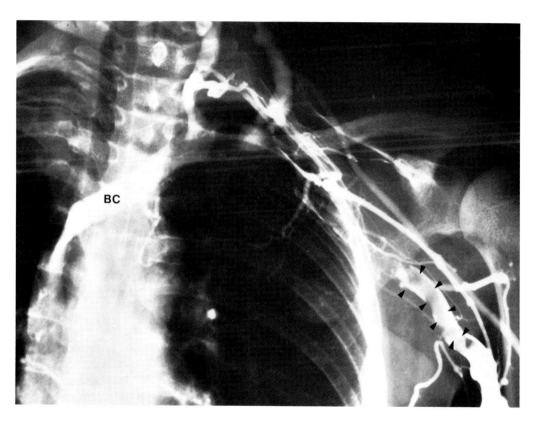

Fig. 19-2. Left upper extremity venography performed for swelling which developed after removal of a central venous catheter demonstrates thrombus in the axillary vein (*arrowheads*) extending into the subclavian vein. Collateral flow through veins in the neck opacifies the brachiocephalic (*BC*) vein.

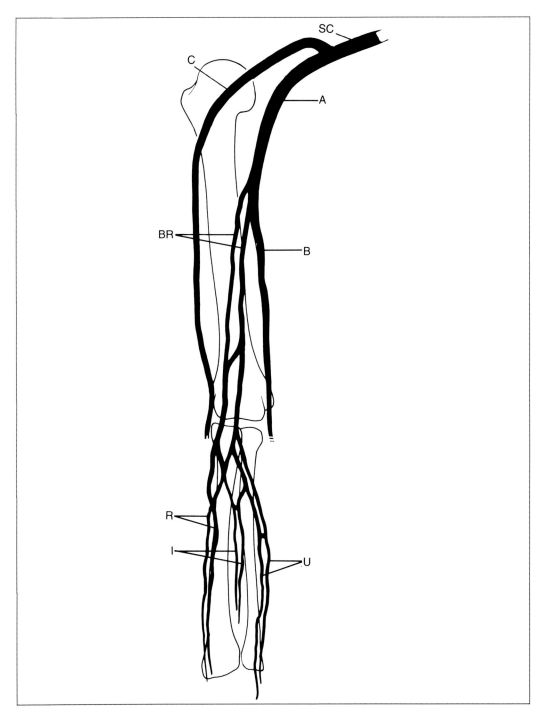

Fig. 19-3. Diagrammatic representation of the veins of the upper extremity. *SC*, subclavian vein; *A*, axillary vein; *C*, cephalic vein; *B*, basilic vein; *BR*, brachial veins; *R*, radial veins; *I*, interosseous veins; *U*, ulnar veins.

20

Inferior Venacavography

Kerry M. Link

Indications:
Inferior venacavography is performed before filter placement and is also indicated for the evaluation of caval occlusion from lower extremity or pelvic extension of venous thrombosis, obstruction as a result of tumor extension (renal cell carcinoma), or compression by other retroperitoneal processes (lymphadenopathy, retroperitoneal fibrosis).

Risks:
In addition to risks associated with venous contrast material administration, there is a risk of hematoma development at the venous access site, especially if the patient is being treated with anticoagulants. There is a small risk of clot migration if a clot is present in the vena cava at the time of contrast material injection.

Catheterization:
Catheterization is performed with a 4 to 5 Fr 60-cm pigtail catheter inserted from a femoral approach. Alternatively, the study may be performed with the pulmonary angiography catheter after pulmonary embolism is documented. A 90-cm catheter length may be necessary if arm access is used.

Injection:
A high iodine concentration contrast material is used (350 mg I/ml). Rates of 15 to 20 cc/s for a total volume of 45 to 80 cc are appropriate. (Routine: 20 cc/s for a total volume of 60 cc).

Filming Sequence:
Single plane:
2 films/s $\times$ 3 s; 1 film/s $\times$ 6 s.

Biplane:
4 films/s $\times$ 3 s; 2 films/s $\times$ 6 s.

Technique: The common femoral vein is usually the safest and most convenient route of entry. The right side is preferred, as entry of the left iliac vein into the inferior vena cava is more obtuse, making catheterization for pulmonary arteriography or filter placement technically more difficult.

The femoral arterial pulse should be continuously palpated. An Amplatz needle (Becton-Dickinson, Franklin Lakes, NJ) with the obturator removed is loaded on a 10-cc syringe filled with 5 cc of saline flush solution and passed into the vein while the patient performs a Valsalva maneuver. The site of venous entry is 2 cm inferior and 1 cm medial to the site normally selected for arterial entry.

Suction is applied to the syringe as the needle is withdrawn. Entry of the needle into the vein is indicated by aspiration of venous blood into the syringe. The sheath portion of the needle is passed into the vein.

To check for common femoral or external iliac vein thrombosis, 10 cc of contrast material is injected rapidly by hand. Spot films at a rate of 4/s can be obtained. If thrombosis is not identified, a standard J guidewire is advanced through the sheath into the lower inferior vena cava. The pigtail catheter is inserted over the guidewire and placed with the tip in the external iliac vein. If thrombus is present, it may be possible to negotiate a catheter beyond this site; alternatively, the contralateral femoral vein may be punctured. If inferior venacavography precedes pulmonary angiography, the venotomy site can then be dilated to 7 to 8 Fr, depending on the catheter of choice. Inferior venacavography can be performed after pulmonary embolus is confirmed in anticipation of vena cava filter placement with the pulmonary angiography catheter; however, the inferior vena cava should be assessed for clot fluoroscopically, before the catheter is passed into the heart.

If Doppler ultrasound or other studies suggest femoral or iliac venous occlusion, an upper extremity approach can be used with puncture of the medial basilic vein. A 90-cm pigtail catheter can be advanced into the inferior vena cava across the right atrium. This approach may also be necessary in assessing the upper extent of inferior vena cava occlusion resulting from renal cell carcinoma extension; this determination has a direct bearing on the choice of operative approach.

One of the most common indications for the performance of this study is to document inferior vena cava anatomy prior to caval filter placement. In these cases, a grid or ruler should be placed below the patient before filming to assure accurate measurement of inferior vena caval diameter. Biplane studies may be helpful to assess the overall configuration of the vessel. In addition to identifying any thrombus, it is imperative to determine the level of the renal venous inflow. This level is identified by the presence of nonopacified blood entering the inferior vena cava in the vicinity of the L1 vertebral body. Occasionally, there is retrograde flow into these vessels.

SUGGESTED READINGS

Lein HH, Kolbenstvedt A: Nonmalignant venographic abnormalities of the inferior vena cava. Radiology 122:105, 1977

Mayo J, Gray R, St. Louis E et al: Anomalies of the inferior vena cava. AJR 140:339, 1983

Prince MR, Novelline RA, Athanasoulis CA, Simon M: The diameter of the inferior vena cava and its implications for the use of vena cava filters. Radiology 149:687, 1983

Selby JB Jr, Pryor JL, Tegtmeyer CJ, Gillenwater JY: Inferior vena caval invasion by renal cell carcinoma: false positive diagnosis by venacavography. J Urol 143:464, 1990

Illustrations

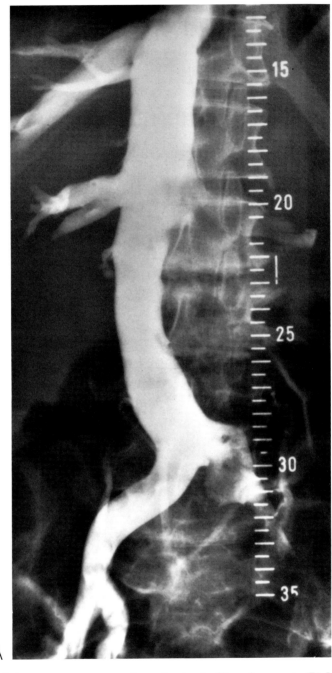

Fig. 20-1. (A) Inferior venacavogram performed prior to filter placement. **(B)** Labeled drawing of inferior vena cava. *RH*, right hepatic vein; *MH*, middle hepatic vein; *RR*, right renal vein; *LR*, left renal vein; *RCI*, right common iliac vein; *LCI*, left common iliac vein; *AscL*, ascending lumbar veins.

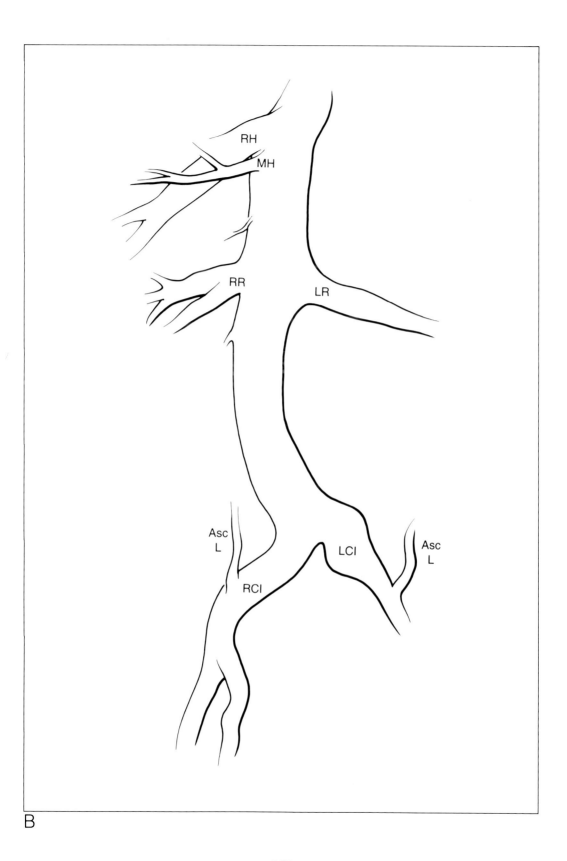

B

165

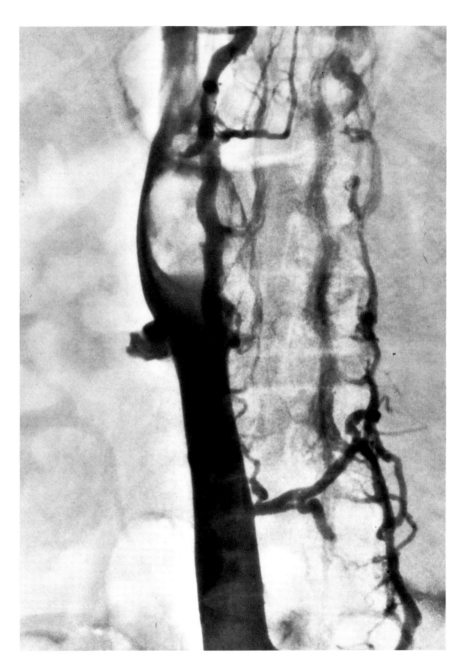

Fig. 20-2. An inferior venacavogram in a patient with a left renal cell carcinoma shows a large filling defect extending from the left renal vein, which represents tumor thrombus. Note the filling of ascending lumbar and epidural veins as collateral channels.

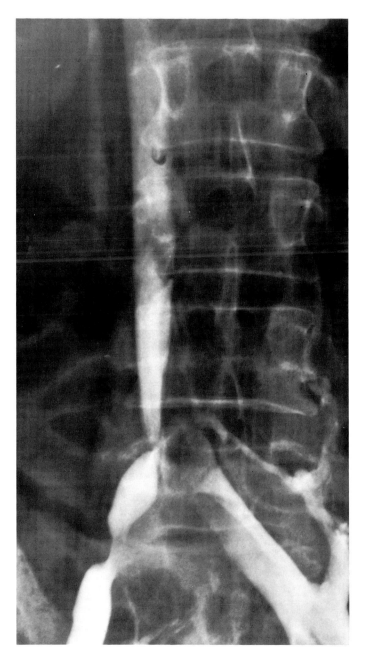

Fig. 20-3. In this patient with retroperitoneal fibrosis, the inferior venacavogram shows compression of the common iliac veins and caudal vena cava resulting from fibrotic plaque.

21

Pulmonary Arteriography

Ray Dyer

Indications: The angiographic study is considered the standard for the diagnosis of pulmonary embolus. It is also used in the evaluation of pulmonary hypertension and the rare pulmonary arteriovenous malformation.

Risks: Venous entry is associated with a slightly lower risk than is arterial entry. The risk of bleeding may be enhanced if the patient is already being treated with anticoagulants at the time of study. In addition to the risk of reaction to contrast material administration, catheter manipulation through the heart may induce cardiac arrhythmias. During passage of the catheter through the heart, a right bundle branch block may be induced, so that a patient with a preexisting left bundle branch block may require prophylactic insertion of a pacemaker to prevent asystole. Patients with high right ventricular end diastolic pressure (>20 mmHg) and high pulmonary artery pressure (>70 mmHg) also are at risk for asystole.

Catheterization: A 7 to 8 Fr pigtail catheter with right angle configuration (Van Aman or Grollman) is preferable.

Injection: A high iodine concentration nonionic contrast agent (350 mg I/ml) is used. Selective right or left pulmonary artery injections are preferred, and rates of 20 to 25 cc/s for a total volume of 40 to 50 cc are employed. (Routine: 25 cc/s for a total volume of 50 cc). Selective segmental artery injection is favored with high pressures or for evaluation of questionable areas. Lower volumes should be used (10 to 20 cc/s for a total volume of 15 to 25 cc).

169

Filming Sequence: Because flow from pulmonary artery to pulmonary vein requires less than 5 s, very rapid filming is necessary unless cardiac output is decreased or pulmonary hypertension is present.

Single plane:
3–4 films/s × 3–4 s; 2 films/s × 2 s; 1 film/s × 4 s.

Biplane sequence (for slowed flow):
4 films/s × 4 s; 2 films/s × 6 s. This sequence yields 2 films/s × 4 s; 1 film/s × 6 s in each plane.

Technique: The chest radiograph and ventilation–perfusion scan, if available, should always be reviewed prior to arteriography. In the unstable patient, a perfusion study may serve to direct angiographic investigation to the area of highest suspicion.

The right common femoral vein is the most convenient site of entry. Venous entry is accomplished as described in Chapter 3. A standard J guidewire is introduced to the level of the iliac vein bifurcation and the venotomy dilated to the appropriate size. The dilator can be left in place and an injection of contrast material monitored fluoroscopically to assure that the inferior vena cava is free of clot. If thrombus is seen, a formal venacavogram should be obtained.

If the passage is not obstructed, the catheter is connected to a pressure monitor. The catheter is manipulated through the heart as pressures are obtained. The electrocardiogram should be monitored continuously during catheter passage. The pigtail is turned medially and directed through the tricuspid valve. The catheter is then rotated and advanced out the pulmonary artery.

Normal Pressures (in mmHg)			
	Systolic	*Diastolic*	*Mean*
Right atrium	0	0	0–5
Right ventricle	20–25	0–7	0
Pulmonary artery	20–25	8–12	15

Particular attention should be paid to patients with right ventricular end diastolic pressure greater than 20 mmHg, which indicates maximal right ventricular afterload and significant risk of asystole with large main pulmonary artery injections. Asystole may also occur with pulmonary artery pressures higher than 70 mmHg systolic. In these cases segmental vessel injection with reduced volumes should be used.

The catheter is positioned in the vessel of highest positive probability as indicated by clinical complaint, radiograph, or ventilation–perfusion study. If an area of reasonable probability is negative on one view, a second view should be obtained. Consideration should also be given to magnification views and superselective arterial injections.

The diagnosis of pulmonary embolus is made by demonstrating vessel cutoff, usually with a convex proximal margin, or an intraluminal filling defect surrounded by contrast. Apparent vessel loss, reduced lung opacification, or slowed flow is not sufficient for angiographic diagnosis.

For selective main right or left pulmonary artery injections the patient is placed in a slight contralateral oblique position to turn the heart off the lower lobe vasculature where emboli are most likely to lodge. (The right pulmonary artery would be studied with the patient in a slight left posterior oblique position.) A second view, usually with the patient in the opposite oblique position, is obtained as needed. The study is continued until pulmonary embolism is found or until all vessels are adequately studied. (A normal perfusion study effectively excludes a clinically significant pulmonary embolus.)

Pulmonary hypertension is defined as a pulmonary artery pressure greater than 30 mmHg systolic.

Mild: 30 to 40 mmHg

Moderate: 40 to 70 mmHg

Severe: greater than 70 mmHg

SUGGESTED READINGS

Alderson PO, Martin EC: Pulmonary embolism: diagnosis with multiple imaging modalities. Radiology 164:297, 1987

Bookstein JJ: Pulmonary thromboembolism with emphasis on angiographic-pathologic correlation. Semin Roentgenol 5:291, 1970

Bookstein JJ, Silver TM: The angiographic differential diagnosis of acute pulmonary embolism. Radiology 110:25, 1974

Johnsrude IS, Jackson DC, Dunnick NR: A Practical Approach to Angiography. 2nd Ed. Little, Brown, Boston, 1987

Mills SR, Jackson DC, Older RA et al: The incidence, etiologies, and avoidance of complications of pulmonary angiography in a large series. Radiology 136:295, 1980

Illustrations

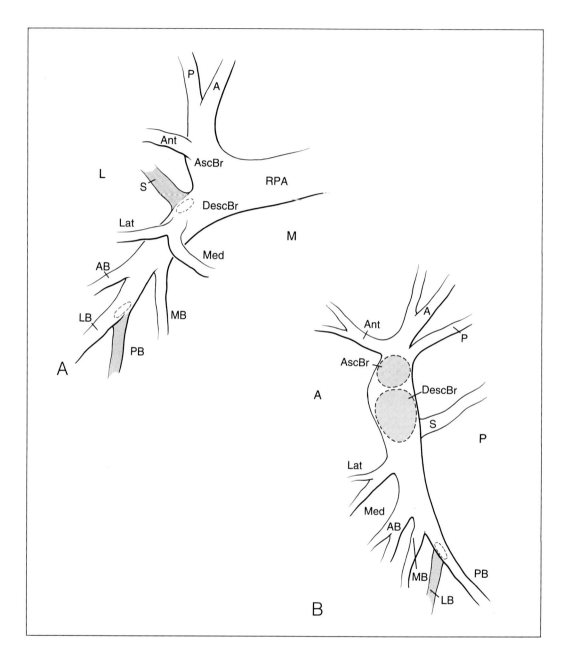

Fig. 21-1. (A & B) Diagrammatic rendering of the right pulmonary artery branches in anteroposterior and lateral views (*A*, anterior; *P*, posterior; *M*, medial; *L*, lateral). *RPA*, right main pulmonary artery; *AscBr*, ascending branch; *DescBr*, descending branch; *A*, apical segmental artery (upper lobe); *P*, posterior segmental artery (upper lobe); *Ant*, anterior segmental artery (upper lobe); *S*, superior segmental artery (lower lobe); *Lat*, lateral segmental artery (middle lobe); *Med*, medial segmental artery (middle lobe); *AB*, anterior basal segmental artery (lower lobe); *LB*, lateral basal segmental artery (lower lobe); *PB*, posterior basal segmental artery (lower lobe); *MB*, medial basal segmental artery (lower lobe).

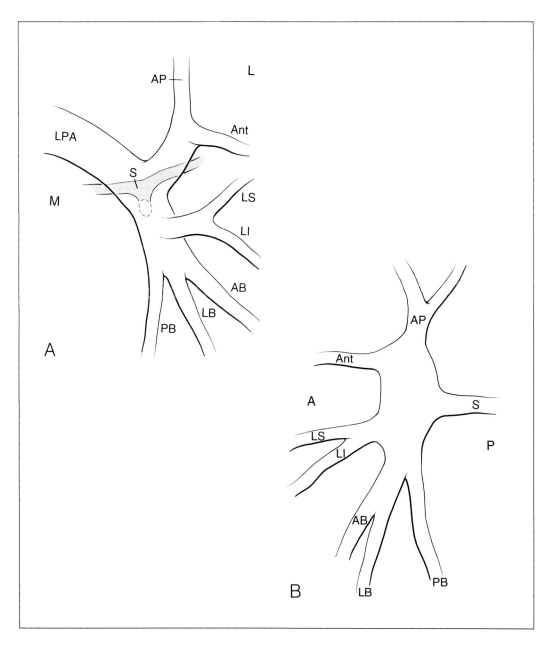

Fig. 21-2. (A & B) Diagrammatic rendering of the left pulmonary artery branches in anteroposterior and lateral views (*A*, anterior; *P*, posterior; *M*, medial; *L*, lateral). *LPA*, left main pulmonary artery; *AP*, apical posterior segmental artery (upper lobe); *Ant*, anterior segmental artery (upper lobe); *S*, superior segmental artery (lower lobe); *LS*, lingular superior segmental artery; *LI*, lingular inferior segmental artery; *AB*, anterior basal segmental artery (lower lobe); *LB*, lateral basal segmental artery (lower lobe); *PB*, posterior basal segmental artery (lower lobe); *, the medial basal segmental artery is rarely seen.

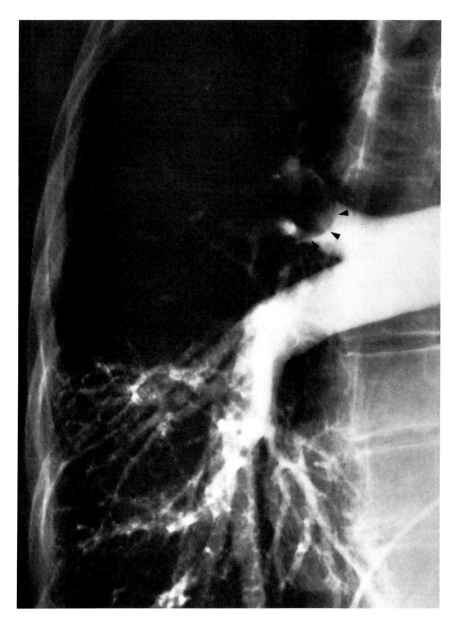

Fig. 21-3. A selective right pulmonary arteriogram demonstrates the convex proximal edge (*arrowheads*) of an embolus occupying the entire ascending branch. Reduced lung opacification distal to the embolus is also seen.

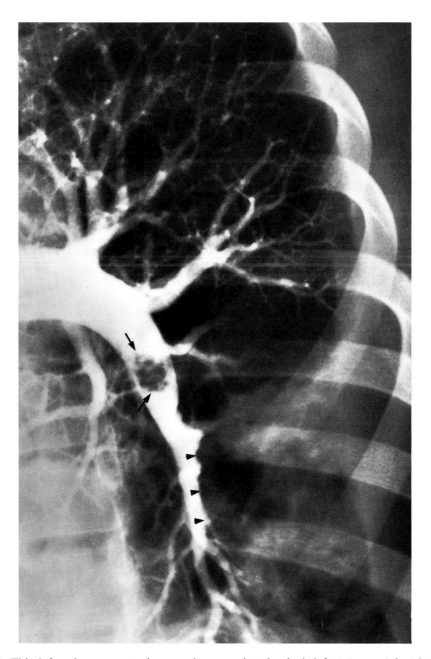

Fig. 21-4. This left pulmonary arteriogram shows an intraluminal defect (*arrows*) just below the takeoff of the lingular segmental vessels. Note the absence of filling of the anterior and lateral basal segmental arteries. Irregularity of the vessel margin (*arrowheads*) represents the proximal end of an embolus that has occluded these vessels.

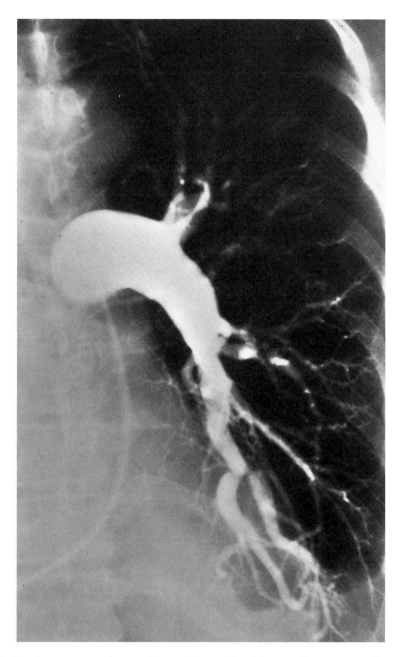

Fig. 21-5. Left pulmonary arteriogram in a patient with a history of recurrent pulmonary emboli shows stenosis at the origins of the posterior and lateral basal segmental arteries. This appearance may be seen after recanalization of a vessel following embolic occlusion.

22

Renal Venography

Kerry M. Link

Indications: Renal venography is performed in the evaluation of renal vein thrombosis, tumor invasion of the renal vein, essential hematuria secondary to renal vein varices, and renal vein abnormalities in transplant donors, in presurgical evaluation and postsurgical follow-up of patients with splenorenal shunts, and in the determination of renin levels in patients with suspected renal vascular hypertension.

Risks: Risks include those associated with venous access and exposure to contrast material. Catheter-induced renal vein thrombosis and dissection are extremely rare.

Catheterization: The preferred approach is via the right common femoral vein. A 6.5 Fr Cobra catheter with multiple side holes is used for general renal venography. For renal vein renin sampling, a 7 Fr sheath is inserted at the puncture site, and two 5.5 Fr Cobra catheters with two side holes are used to catheterize the left and right renal veins individually and simultaneously (see below).

Injection: An intermediate iodine concentration contrast agent is used (300 mg I/ml). For general renal venography, 8 cc/s for a total volume of 25 cc is used. For renal vein renin acquisition, contrast material is injected by hand into each vein to document appropriate catheter position after sample acquisition.

Filming Sequence: *Renal venography:*
3–4 films/s × 5 s.

Renal vein renin catheter documentation:
Spot films at 2 films/s.

Technique: The right common femoral vein is cannulated as described in Chapter 3. A 6.5 Fr Cobra catheter is introduced into the inferior vena cava to the level of the T12–L1 disc space. The catheter is withdrawn until the vein of interest is engaged. On the left, the catheter tip is placed as far as possible into the main renal vein in an effort to potentiate reflux into the intrarenal veins and to avoid reflux into the gonadal vein. Good opacification will avoid potential pitfalls in diagnosis produced by nonopacified gonadal vein blood entering into the proximal aspect of the renal vein. This process can mimic thrombosis or tumor.

For formal renal venography, a 6-in. magnification view coned to include the kidney and the anticipated inferior vena cava insertion site is obtained, using a small focal spot. For documentation of catheter position, a 6-in. magnification spot film is obtained and coned to include the kidney of interest and the inferior vena cava.

Because of the extremely high blood flow in both the arterial and venous sides of the renal vasculature, it is important to inject high doses of contrast material at a rapid rate to opacify the renal venous system. Very commonly, renal venography is performed in conjunction with renal artery evaluation. In such cases, epinephrine (10 μg) can be injected into the renal artery via the arterial catheter prior to renal venography to decrease the rapid flow through the kidney. As a result, the ability to opacify the entire venous system is enhanced. It should be noted, however, that for studying patients with renal cell tumors and possible tumor extension into the renal vein, epinephrine is not usually beneficial, as tumor vessels are less reponsive to epinephrine than normal vessels.

For evaluation of renal transplant donors, renal venography is usually not required. Selective renal artery injection will suffice if on the delayed films the veins are identified. However, anatomic abnormalities, such as the circumaortic renal vein, may impact on renal harvesting and should be noted.

When renal venous studies are performed for renal vein renin sampling, the preprocedural evaluation of the patient, patient preparation, and the actual catheterization are modified in the following manner.

1. All beta blockers and angiotensin-converting enzyme inhibitors should be discontinued at least 3 days prior to the examination, if at all possible.
2. Furosemide (40 mg) should be administered orally the evening before the examination.
3. The patient should have nothing by mouth and intravenous

fluids should be limited to a keep-open rate, using fluids without sodium content.

4. The patient should be kept supine for 3 h prior to performance of the study.

5. When being transferred to the examination table, the patient should be kept supine.

6. After cannulation of the right common femoral vein, a 7 Fr sheath should be introduced. This sheath will accept two 0.35-in. guidewires, and upon removal of the sheath, two 5.5 Fr Cobra catheters, each with two side holes, can be inserted over the guidewires to catheterize the right and left renal veins simultaneously. Before placement of the catheters, one inferior vena cava blood sample should be obtained below the level of inflow of the renal veins. The catheters should then be placed in the right and left renal veins. The catheters are left in place for 10 min, after which time three sets of bilateral renal vein blood samples are obtained simultaneously at 2-min intervals. Contrast material is injected into the catheters by hand and spot films are obtained as described above to document catheter position. Finally, an additional inferior vena cava blood sample is obtained below the renal veins after renal vein sampling is completed.

To optimize the examination regardless of the reason for its performance, an adequate understanding of renal vein anatomy is essential. Valves are often encountered within the renal veins. They occur in 28% to 70% of the population in the right renal vein and in 4% to 36% of the population in the left renal vein.

With regard to the right system, a single renal vein occurs in 85% of the population. A single renal vein that bifurcates so that it has two insertions to the inferior vena cava occurs in 4% of cases. In 15% of the population, two to four renal veins coexist. On the right side, the gonadal vein joins the right renal vein in 6% of the population. Valves are present in the right gonadal vein in 77% of men and 94% of women. The retroperitoneal veins drain into the right renal vein in only 3% of cases. These draining veins may efflux nonopacified blood, thereby mimicking tumor or thrombosis formation in the main renal vein.

On the left, a single preaortic vein occurs in 86% of the population. A single retroaortic vein occurs in 2.4%, whereas a circumaortic vein occurs in 7%. Multiple renal veins on the left are rare, occurring in only 1% of the population. Retroperitoneal veins, including the lumbar, ascending lumbar, and hemiazygous veins, drain into the left renal vein in 75% of the population. The ureteric vein drains into the intrahilar portion of the renal vein. On the left, multiple draining gonadal veins occur in 15% of people but usually do not number more than two. Valves are noted in the gonadal vein in 60% of men and 86% of women.

SUGGESTED READINGS

Ahlberg NE, Bartley O, Chidekel N: Right and left gonadal veins, an anatomical and statistical study. Acta Radiol 4:593, 1966

Ahlberg N–E, Bartley O, Chidekel N: Occurrence of valves in the main trunk of the renal vein. Acta Radiol 7:431, 1968

Anatkow J, Kumanow C: Selective nephro-phlebography. In Diethelm L (ed): Symposium of the European Association of Radiology. Springer, Mainz, 1972

Hollinshead WH: Renovascular anatomy. Postgrad Med 40:241, 1966

Janower ML: Nephrotic syndrome secondary to renal vein thrombosis. The value of inferior vena cavography. AJR 95:330, 1965

Olin TB, Reuter SR: A pharmacoangiographic method for improving nephrophlebography. Radiology 85:1036, 1965

Pick JW, Anson BJ: The renal vascular pedicle: anatomical study of 430 body-halves. J Urol 44:411, 1940

Reis RH, Esenther G: Variations in the pattern of renal vessels and their relation to the type of posterior vena cava in man. Am J Anat 104:295, 1959

Takaro T, Dow JA, Kishev S: Selective occlusive renal phlebography in man. Radiology 94:589, 1970

Illustrations

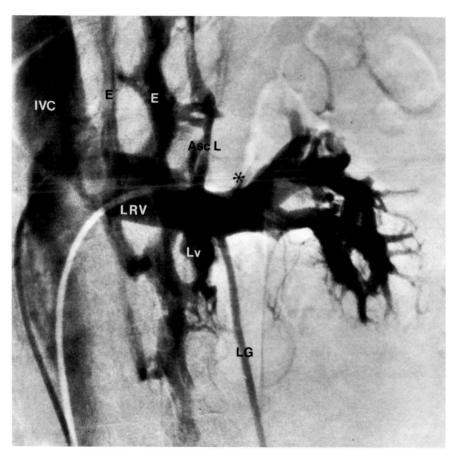

Fig. 22-1. Normal left renal venogram. *IVC*, inferior vena cava; *LRV*, left renal vein; *LV*, lumbar veins; *LG*, left gonadal vein; *AscL*, ascending lumbar vein; *E*, epidural veins; *, adrenal vein inflow.

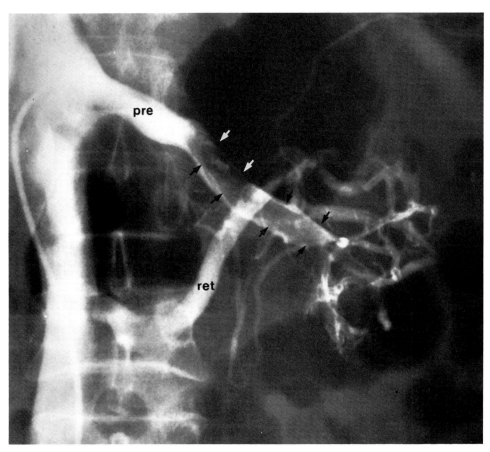

Fig. 22-2. Left renal venography in a patient with amyloidosis who developed nephrotic syndrome shows a circumaortic renal vein, the preaortic limb (*pre*) of which contains a large thrombus (*arrows*). The retroaortic limb (*ret*) enters the inferior vena cava at the L3 level.

23

Lower Extremity Venography

Kerry M. Link

Indications:	Evaluation of the lower extremity venous system is one of the most common venographic procedures. It is frequently used for evaluation of leg swelling specifically associated with deep venous thrombosis and may be used in the evaluation of incompetent perforating veins prior to vein stripping.
Risks:	Procedural risks include reaction to contrast material, contrast material extravasation with tissue damage, post-study phlebitis or thrombosis, and, rarely, periprocedural pulmonary embolism.
Catheterization:	A 21- or 19-gauge butterfly needle is placed distally and medially into a vein on the dorsum of the foot, preferably in the vein to the great toe. A more proximal position on the foot may produce injection directly into the superficial venous arch and result in nonfilling of the deep veins.
Injection:	A low iodine concentration nonionic contrast agent (240 mg I/ml) or an equivalent dilution is injected by hand at a rate of 1 cc/s for a total volume of 150 to 180 cc.
Filming Sequence:	*Lower leg (ankle to below knee):* 14 × 17-in. film lengthwise; 3-on-1 filming—anteroposterior, internal rotation, external rotation. If the leg is large or very edematous, 2-on-1 filming may be necessary. *Centered on knee:* 14 × 17-in. film lengthwise; 3-on-1 filming—anteroposterior, internal rotation, external rotation. If the leg is large or very edematous, 2-on-1 filming may be necessary.

Thigh:
14 × 17-in. film lengthwise; 2-on-1 filming—anteroposterior, external rotation.

Centered on hip:
14 × 17-in. film crosswise; 2-on-1 filming—anteroposterior, external rotation.

Pelvis:
14 × 17-in. film crosswise; 2-on-1 filming—rapid filming sequence.

Technique: The patient is placed on a tilting table with a block underneath the extremity that is *not* to be evaluated. Ensuring that the leg of interest is not weight-bearing increases the venous capacitance, improves filling, and prevents compression of veins by muscular contraction. An abdominal binder assists in supporting the patient when the table is tilted.

The table is tilted 30° above horizontal to pool blood in the foot as an aid to venipuncture, preferably of the medial vein of the great toe or of a vein on the distal half of the foot. Associated edema or the presence of dark skin may cause difficulty in identifying and puncturing a vein. When edema is present, gentle massage of the dorsum of the foot can occasionally accentuate a vein. A fiber-optic light can also assist in identifying a vein. Additional devices that aid in the identification and engorgement of the vein include warm compresses applied to the foot, a blood pressure cuff placed on the calf, an elastic wrap started at the calf and wrapped progressively tighter toward the foot, and nitroglycerin paste applied to the dorsum of the foot. After the vein is identified and prepared for venipuncture, a 21-gauge butterfly needle or, if possible, a 19-gauge butterfly needle is used to cannulate the vein.

There are partial valves between the superficial and deep venous systems of the foot, unlike the complete valves of the leg. The resulting free communication between the superficial and deep venous systems in the region of the distal half of the foot explains the rationale behind the venipuncture in the region of the great toe. Once in place, the butterfly needle should be secured to the patient's skin to avoid dislodgement or venous injury. If venipuncture is unsuccessful, or if after puncture the needle is dislodged, it is important to leave the needle in place to prevent extravasation of contrast material through the venipuncture site.

The table is elevated to approximately 45° and contrast medium is slowly injected by hand. Contrast material should be available in three 60-cc syringes. During the initial period of infusion, fluoroscopy of the foot should be performed in an effort to detect extravasation as early as possible. Through the course of the examination, the foot should be reevaluated occasionally for ex-travasation, and the patient should be asked to report any pain at the site of cannulation.

After infusion of 80 cc of contrast material, the leg is imaged fluoroscopically. If the deep venous system has filled, leg filming is undertaken from a distal-to-proximal direction. It is important to continue constant infusion during filming and to perform the examination quickly to prevent loss of contrast opacification of the venous system. The venous capacitance of the lower extremity is approximately 300 to 700 ml, and a total injection of approxi-mately 120 to 180 cc of contrast material is required for adequate opacification.

If the deep venous system is not successfully demonstrated ini-tially, a tourniquet is placed at the level of the ankle to augment passage of contrast material into the deep venous system of the foot. If this strategy is also unsuccessful, an additional tourniquet can be placed at the level of the calf. It is important to be aware of potential artifacts produced by the presence of the tourniquet.

The examination is temporarily suspended after films have been obtained of the lower leg, knee, thigh, and hip. If film quality is adequate for diagnosis, the patient is then taught how to perform a Valsalva maneuver on command and is instructed to do so while the table is rapidly brought back to the horizontal position. The patient is asked to relax once in the horizontal position. Relaxation of the Valsalva maneuver after rapid leveling of the table should flood the iliac vein and distal inferior vena cava with contrast material from the leg. Rapid filming of the pelvis and lower abdo-men in the anteroposterior projection is then performed as de-scribed above.

Immediately after the exam has been completed, the venous sys-tem should be flushed with intravenous fluids through the foot cannula to wash out residual contrast material from the venous system. This process should prevent the postphlebography syn-drome, which may result from prolonged contact of contrast mate-rial with the venous walls.

The patient's foot should be carefully evaluated during injection for extravasation of contrast material. If extravasation occurs at any time during the examination, infusion is halted and cold compresses are applied to the area. The residual contrast material may be manually expressed through the puncture site. The clinical service should be notified of this complication and foot elevation ordered. Serious extravasation, particularly of ionic contrast materials, can result in significant tissue injury. The radiologist therefore is obliged to check the patient on a daily basis.

The sine qua non for diagnosis of acute deep venous thrombosis is evidence of contrast material around an intraluminal filling defect, sometimes producing a "railroad track" appearance. Indirect evidence of deep venous thrombosis includes abrupt termination of an opacified vein, nonfilling of a portion of the deep venous system, or the presence of collateral venous flow. It should be noted that these three signs are indicative of venous disease, but not necessarily of acute deep venous thrombosis. Irregularity of an opacified vessel and/or reduplication of the venous system is consistent with recanalization and, therefore, of chronic deep venous thrombosis.

Injected air bubbles, underfilling of the venous system from too slow an injection or insufficient patient elevation, and layering and mixing artifacts are all potential causes of filling defects that may cause misdiagnoses. Compression artifacts secondary to muscular contraction, soft tissue hematoma, or a mass such as a popliteal cyst, as well as iatrogenic nonfilling caused by tourniquets, may also cause diagnostic difficulty.

SUGGESTED READINGS

Bettmann MA, Paulin S: Leg phlebography: the incidence, nature and modification of undesirable side effects. Radiology 122:101, 1977

Elam EA, Dorr RT, Lagel KE, Pond GD: Cutaneous ulceration due to contrast extravasation. Experimental assessment of injury and potential antidotes. Invest Radiol 26:13, 1991

Lea Thomas M: Phlebography of the Lower Limb. Churchill Livingstone, New York, 1982

Rabinov K, Paulin S: Roentgen diagnosis of venous thrombosis in the leg. Arch Surg 104:134, 1972

Illustrations

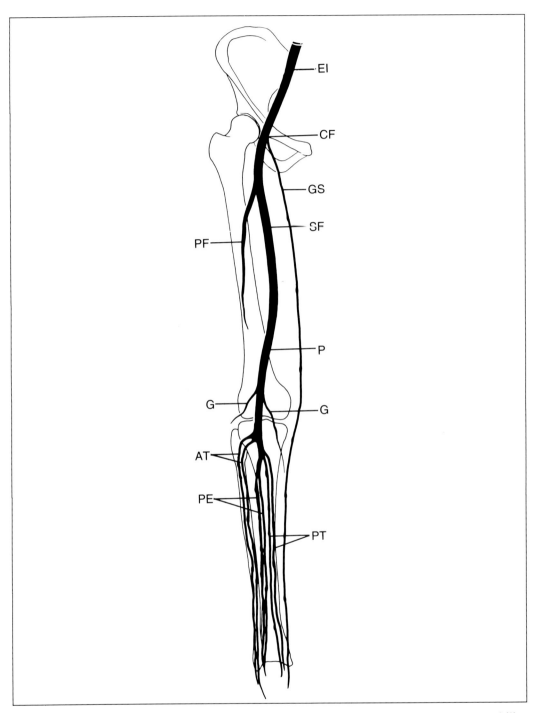

Fig. 23-1. Diagrammatic representation of the deep veins of the lower extremity. *EI*, external iliac vein; *CF*, common femoral vein; *GS*, greater saphenous vein; *PF*, profunda femoris (deep femoral) vein; *SF*, superficial femoral vein; *P*, popliteal vein; *G*, gastrocnemius veins; *AT*, anterior tibial veins; *PE*, peroneal veins; *PT*, posterior tibial veins.

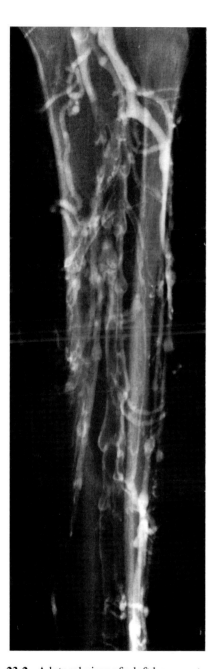

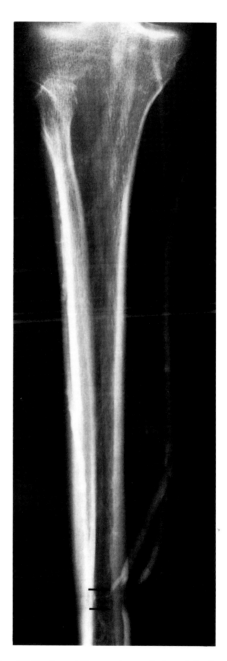

Fig. 23-2. A lateral view of a left lower extremity venogram in a patient with acute calf swelling demonstrates extensive filling defects in the peroneal and posterior tibial veins, giving a "railroad track" appearance, indicative of acute deep venous thrombosis.

Fig. 23-3. An oblique view of the right lower extremity during venography shows no filling of the deep veins of the calf despite the presence of a tourniquet. Note the artifactual compression defect on the saphenous vein (*arrows*). If the superficial venous system has not been injected directly, this finding usually indicates extensive venous thrombosis in the acute setting.

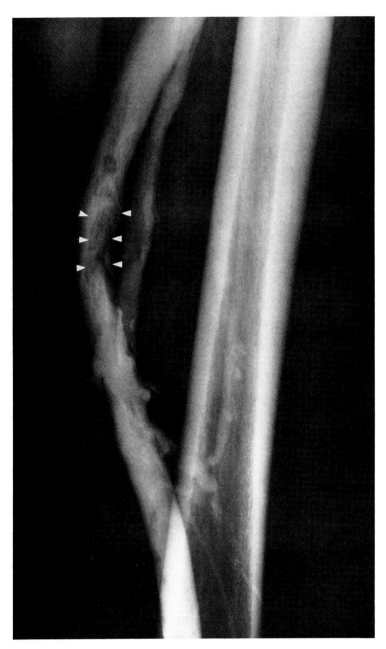

Fig. 23-4. An apparent filling defect (*arrowheads*) is seen in the superficial femoral vein during venography. This defect changed over time, indicating that it is a flow artifact probably created by a valve.

24

Portal Hypertension Evaluation

Kerry M. Link
William P. Jones

Indications: The evaluation of portal hypertension, which consists of assessment of the hepatic veins with venous pressure measurements, and opacification of the portal vein after injection of contrast material into the arterial circulation (arterial portography), is used in the evaluation of portal hypertension in anticipation of portosystemic shunting, or in the follow-up of this procedure. This evaluation may be undertaken prior to liver transplantation. Hepatic venography may also be used to evaluate hepatic venous obstruction (Budd–Chiari syndrome).

Risks: The study requires both venous and arterial access, as well as contrast administration, with the attendant risks. Hepatic venography carries the specific risks of perforation of the liver capsule with a guidewire, catheter, or overzealous wedge injection that may result in intraperitoneal hemorrhage. Excessive injection with a catheter in the wedged position may also produce hemorrhagic hepatic infarction. The risks associated with the arteriographic portions of the evaluation are outlined in the respective sections.

Catheterization: Hepatic venous catheterization is performed with a 7 Fr 80-cm Cobra balloon occlusion catheter with a 12-mm diameter latex occlusion balloon. If the procedure cannot be performed successfully with this catheter, a 65-cm simple-curve endhole catheter may be positioned with the use of a deflector wire. Renal venography and arterial portions of the evaluation are performed as outlined in their respective sections.

Injection: An intermediate iodine concentration contrast material is used for the venographic evaluation (300 mg I/ml). With the catheter in a wedged position, indicated by absence of venous outflow with test injection of 1 cc of contrast material, an injection rate of 1 to 2 cc/s for a total volume of 8 to 10 cc is used. With the catheter in a nonwedged position in the main hepatic or second-order tributary vein, an injection rate of 7 to 10 cc/s for a total volume of 20 to 25 cc is utilized.

Injection rates for the renal venogram and arteriographic portions of the study are outlined in their respective sections.

Filming Sequence: *Catheter in wedged position:*
1 film/s × 12 s. Filming should extend 5 to 10 s after the end of the injection.

Catheter in nonwedged position:
2 film/s × 3 s; 1 film/s × 3 s.

See the section on renal venography and appropriate arteriography sections for filming sequences for these studies. The arterial filming sequences should be extended for 30 s to assure venous opacification.

Technique: The evaluation of portal hypertension and delineation of portal venous anatomy require separate venous and arterial access. The femoral route is preferred. Venous evaluation can be accomplished from a right internal jugular approach if the femoral route is compromised.

Hepatic venography with venous pressure measurements:
Once venous access is established, a standard J guidewire is introduced into the inferior vena cava. A 7 Fr Cobra balloon occlusion catheter is introduced to a point just inferior to the diaphragm. The hepatic veins enter the inferior vena cava at this level. The catheter is used to engage a hepatic vein, and a guidewire is advanced toward the periphery of the liver. The catheter is then advanced over the guidewire. Care should be taken to monitor any resistance to passage of the catheter or guidewire to prevent inadvertent hepatic perforation.

The catheter tip is placed in a wedged position, indicated by absence of venous outflow around the catheter with test injection. If the balloon occlusion catheter cannot be passed into a wedged position, inflation of the occlusion balloon and pressure measurement will closely approximate a wedged pressure.

If appropriate measurements cannot be obtained with the Cobra catheter, a simple right-angle curved catheter with an end hole can often be positioned in the hepatic vein over a tip deflector guidewire. The catheter is used to engage the hepatic venous orifice, and the tip deflector guidewire is advanced into the catheter and curved to maintain the position of the catheter at the orifice of the hepatic vein. The catheter is then advanced over the deflector wire into a wedged position. Care should be taken that the tip of the deflector wire never extends beyond the tip of the catheter.

At least two wedge measurements should be obtained, preferably from two separate veins. In addition, a pressure is obtained with the catheter tip free within a large hepatic vein. The catheter is then withdrawn into the inferior vena cava, where another pressure is obtained. In the evaluation of hepatic venous obstruction, right atrial and infrahepatic inferior vena cava pressures should also be obtained.

The hepatic wedge pressure (HWP) corresponds closely to the portal vein pressure. HWP has two components: the hepatic sinusoidal pressure and the intra-abdominal pressure. To determine the hepatic sinusoidal pressure, which represents the degree of obstruction to portal flow by hepatic disease, a corrected sinusoidal pressure (CSP) is calculated. This pressure is obtained by subtracting the free hepatic venous pressure (FHV), which reflects the intra-abdominal pressure, from the HWP.

$$CSP = HWP - FHV$$

Normal Pressures (mmHg)
HWP < 10
FHV < 5
CSP ≤ 5

Severity of cirrhosis can be classified on the basis of the CSP.

Severity of Cirrhosis Based on CSP Measurement (mmHg)
Normal ≤ 5
Mild 6–10
Moderate 11–18
Severe ≥ 19

When the hepatic venous studies and pressure measurements are completed, the catheter is positioned in the left renal vein, and left renal venography is performed. This is done to evaluate for anatomic abnormalities such as a retroaortic or circumaortic renal vein, which could complicate splenorenal decompressive shunts. Following venography, the catheter is left in this position to demarcate the left renal vein during opacification of the splenic and portal veins while arterial portography is performed.

Arterial Portography:
Femoral artery access is established, and a standard J guidewire is advanced into the abdominal aorta. Liver panangiography is performed to evaluate the hepatic arterial system for evidence of cirrhosis and to exclude associated abnormalities, including tumors such as hepatoma, which have an increased incidence in patients with cirrhosis. Splenic artery catheterization is performed for indirect angiographic evaluation of the splenic and portal vein. If opacification of the splenic and portal venous anatomy is inadequate, direct splenoportography or transhepatic portal catheterization may be performed. These procedures are more invasive and are beyond the scope of this handbook.

Once the splenic vein is opacified, the relationship between the splenic vein and the left renal vein (demarcated by the catheter left in place after the venous studies) is documented on film.

Superior mesenteric arteriography (see Ch. 12) is then performed with late-phase filming for evaluation of the mesenteric and portal veins. Opacification of the mesenteric and portal veins may be enhanced with the use of vasodilators (papaverine, tolazoline).

STEPWISE EVALUATION OF PORTAL HYPERTENSION

(*Summary*)

1. Femoral venous access is obtained, and a 7 Fr Cobra balloon occlusion catheter is introduced.
2. A peripheral hepatic vein is catheterized.
3. A wedged hepatic venous pressure is obtained.
4. A free hepatic venous pressure is obtained.
5. Steps 3 and 4 are repeated at a second hepatic venous site.
6. Pressure is obtained in the inferior vena cava.
7. Pressure is obtained in the right atrium.
8. Pressure is obtained in the infrahepatic inferior vena cava.
9. The left renal vein is catheterized.
10. A left renal venogram is performed. Renal vein and local inferior vena cava pressures are obtained if a retroaortic or circumaortic vein is present.
11. The venous catheter is secured in position in the left renal vein during the performance of the arterial study.
12. The femoral artery is entered, and a 5 to 5.5 Fr RC catheter is introduced.
13. Survey celiac arteriography is performed (see Ch. 8).
14. Selective common hepatic artery catheterization and arteriography are performed (see Ch. 9).
15. A selective splenic artery injection with late-phase filming is

performed if the splenic and portal vein are not sufficiently visualized from the celiac artery injection.

16. Superior mesenteric arteriography with late-phase filming is performed for opacification of the mesenteric and portal vein (see Ch. 12).

17. The relationship between the splenic vein and the left renal vein as indicated by the renal venous catheter is established and documented.

SUGGESTED READINGS

Groszmann RJ, Glickman M, Blei AT et al: Wedged and free hepatic venous pressure measured with a balloon catheter. Gastroenterology 76:253, 1979

Johnsrude IS, Jackson DC, Dunnick NR: A Practical Approach to Angiography. 2nd Ed. Little, Brown, Boston, 1987

Kadir S: Diagnostic Angiography. WB Saunders, Philadelphia, 1986

Nordlinger BM, Nordlinger DF, Fulenwider JT et al: Angiography in portal hypertension. Clinical significance in surgery. Am J Surg 139:132, 1980

Pollard JJ, Nebesar RA: Catheterization of the splenic artery for portal venography. N Engl J Med 271:234, 1964

Tisnado J, Cho S-R, Carithers RL Jr et al: The Budd Chiari syndrome: angiographic pathologic correlation. Radiographics 3:155, 1983

Viallet A, Joly J-G, Marleau D, Lavoie P: Comparison of free portal venous pressure and wedged hepatic venous pressure in patients with cirrhosis of the liver. Gastroenterology 59:372, 1970

Viamonte M Jr, Warren WD, Fomon JJ: Liver panangiography in the assessment of portal hypertension in liver cirrhosis. Radiol Clin North Am 8:147, 1970

Widrich WC, Nordahl DL, Robbins AH: Contrast enhancement of the mesenteric and portal veins using intra-arterial papaverine. AJR 121:374, 1974

Illustrations

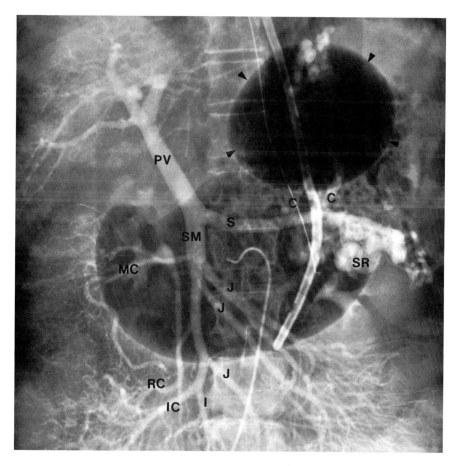

Fig. 24-1. Arterial portography after superior mesenteric artery injection with tolazoline (25 mg) augmentation in a patient with cirrhosis and massive upper gastrointestinal bleeding shows retrograde flow in the splenic vein and filling of gastric and esophageal varices. The inflated gastric balloon (*arrowheads*) of a Sengstaken–Blakemore tube is in the gastric fundus. *PV*, portal vein; *SM*, superior mesenteric vein; *S*, splenic vein; *C*, coronary (left gastric) vein; *MC*, middle colic vein; *RC*, right colic vein; *IC*, ileocolic vein; *I*, ileal vein; *J*, jejunal veins; *SR*, splenoretroperitoneal collateral vein.

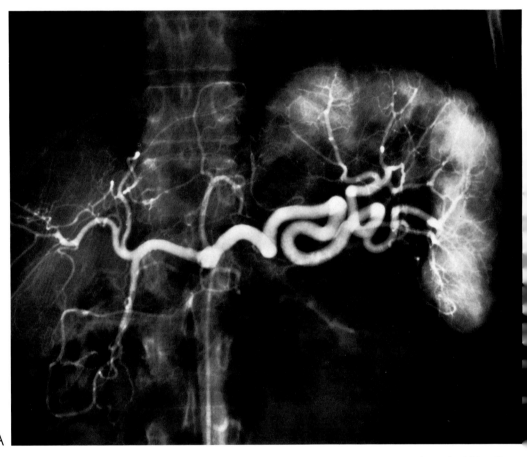

A

Fig. 24-2. (A) Celiac arteriography performed for evaluation of acute upper gastrointestinal bleeding shows no abnormality. (*Figure continues*).

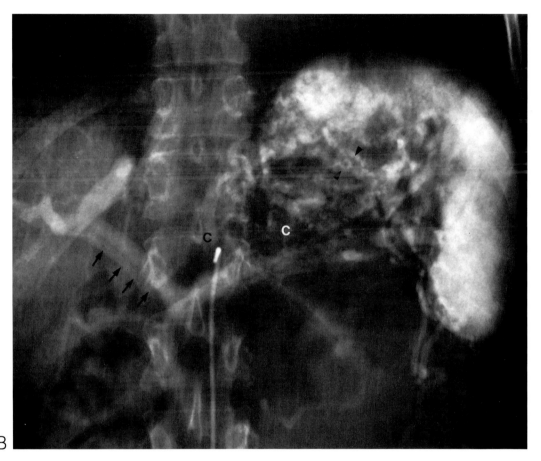

B

Fig. 24-2 (*Continued*). **(B)** Late filming shows irregular filling defects in the splenic vein, a consequence of recanalization. Collateral flow through short gastric veins (*arrowheads*) and coronary veins (*C*) is seen. Note the pseudothrombus from unopacified superior mesenteric venous inflow (*arrows*) in the portal vein.

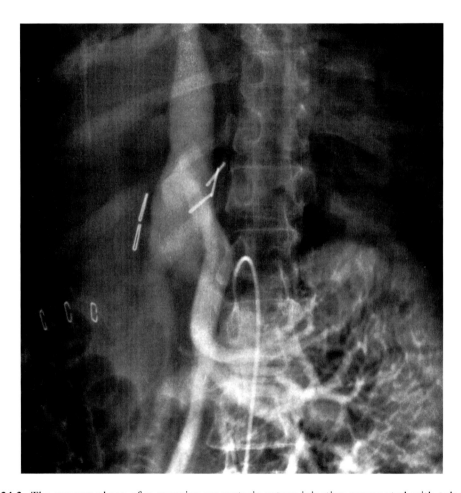

Fig. 24-3. The venous phase of a superior mesenteric artery injection augmented with tolazoline (25 mg) documents patency of a mesocaval shunt created for decompression of esophageal varices.

25

Percutaneous Transluminal Angioplasty

William D. Routh

ILIAC ANGIOPLASTY

Indications:
The indications for angioplasty in the iliac vessels include lifestyle-limiting claudication or resting ischemia caused by stenosis. The procedure is also performed to improve inflow prior to planned femoral–femoral or femoral–distal lower extremity surgical revascularization.

Risks:
Angiographic evaluation prior to angioplasty is necessary for therapeutic planning and carries the attendant risks associated with vascular entry and exposure to contrast material. The angioplasty procedure carries the risk of occlusive arterial dissection, acute thrombosis, distal embolization, or arterial rupture.

Technique:
Femoral artery entry ipsilateral to the iliac stenosis to be dilated is favored and may require cannulation of a nonpalpable artery, as described in Chapter 3. For lesions of the distal external iliac or common femoral artery, and in patients with a favorable aortic bifurcation, the contralateral femoral artery approach may be employed. If ipsilateral femoral entry is possible, a standard J guidewire is used for vessel entry. The wire is advanced into the iliac artery but is kept a few centimeters distal to the area of the stenosis to avoid vessel dissection. Placement of an arterial introducer sheath (6 Fr inner diameter) may facilitate catheter manipulation and prevent vessel trauma with multiple catheter exchanges.

A 5 Fr angle-tipped catheter (JB-1) is inserted over the guidewire or through the vascular sheath. The J guidewire is removed, and contrast material is injected by hand to define the stenotic lesion. Digital roadmapping may be used to provide a real-time fluoroscopic image of the stenosis. A Bentson guidewire can usually be directed through the stenosis with the JB-1 catheter. A steerable guidewire (TAD wire or Glidewire) may be necessary for difficult lesions. The TAD wire is less likely to cause vessel dissection than is the Glidewire and is more stable for catheter exchanges (Fig. 25-1A).

Once the catheter has been negotiated through the lesion into the aorta, an intraarterial bolus of heparin (40 IU/kg) is given. A 4 to 5 Fr pigtail catheter is inserted for performance of preangioplasty pelvic arteriography if this has not been previously performed (see Ch. 14). Pressure should be measured in the aorta and external iliac artery distal to the stenosis. This procedure is facilitated by the presence of a vascular introducer sheath. Angiograms are reviewed and the appropriate sized angioplasty balloon selected. A balloon angioplasty catheter with a 5 Fr shaft is used in most circumstances. A larger caliber catheter may be required for balloon diameters of 10 mm or greater. The diameter of the inflated balloon is selected to match the direct measurement of the opacified luminal diameter of the "normal" vessel adjacent to the stenosis, without correction for filming magnification.

The pigtail catheter is withdrawn over a guidewire, and the angioplasty balloon is inserted (Fig. 25-1B). An inflation handle with an in-line pressure gauge (LeVeen inflator, Medi-tech, Watertown, MA) is used to slowly inflate the angioplasty balloon with contrast material, under constant fluoroscopic observation. A waist-like indentation is often noted in the balloon at the site of the stenosis, as inflation proceeds. With inflation to maximal diameter, this waist should be eliminated (Fig. 25-1C). There is no proven value of applying additional balloon pressure beyond this point. The manufacturer's recommended balloon inflation pressure should not be exceeded.

The balloon is initially inflated for approximately 45 s and then deflated to allow reperfusion. The balloon is reinflated to see if the waist persists. If the waist remains, dilatation may be inadequate, and a larger balloon may be necessary. If no waist is detected, the angioplasty catheter is exchanged over a guidewire for a pigtail catheter and postangioplasty pelvic arteriography is performed. Pressure measurements proximal and distal to the lesion are also repeated.

Catheter–guidewire access through the lesion is never abandoned until follow-up films are carefully reviewed and the patient is clinically stable. A satisfactory result is indicated by pressure measurement proximal and distal to the stenosis with less than a 10-mm systolic gradient and no angiographic evidence of a complication, including obstructing dissection, vessel thrombosis, or rupture. A pigtail catheter should be straightened over a guidewire and removed to prevent trauma to the dilated segment, and the puncture site is compressed to achieve hemostasis.

Postangioplasty care is similar to that for other diagnostic angiographic procedures except for the addition of low-dose aspirin as a platelet aggregation inhibitor. Ambulation is begun the next day, and noninvasive laboratory studies, including segmental pressures and pulse volume recordings, are obtained before discharge.

Management of Complications: Obstructing vessel dissection is initially treated by repeat balloon inflation. In the near future, expandable intravascular metallic stents will be generally available for this indication. Thrombosis at the angioplasty site or distal embolization may require thrombolytic therapy.

Vessel rupture, seen angiographically as contrast extravasation or pseudoaneurysm formation, is controlled by immediate reinflation of the angioplasty balloon to tamponade the bleeding site. Emergency vascular surgical consultation is a necessity. Treatment options for angioplasty-related iliac artery rupture include direct surgical repair or transcatheter coil occlusion of the injured vessel followed by extraanatomic surgical bypass grafting. Anecdotal cases of definitive treatment of the iliac artery rupture by prolonged balloon tamponade have been described.

Results: Initial technical success for iliac artery angioplasty exceeds 90%. A compilation of data from multiple series totaling over 2,500 iliac angioplasty procedures reveals a mean 2-yr patency rate of 81% (range, 65% to 93%) and a mean 5-yr patency rate of 72% (range, 50% to 86%). Long segment iliac stenoses, iliac occlusions, and eccentric stenoses generally respond less favorably to angioplasty than do short segment (<3 cm) concentric stenoses. Iliac angioplasty has similar patency rates to aortobifemoral bypass grafting and eliminates the risk of operative mortality (2% to 3% with similar patency rates) (Figs. 25-2).

RENAL ANGIOPLASTY

Indications: Renal artery angioplasty is usually considered for the hypertensive patient with angiographically demonstrable renal artery stenosis. In patients with unilateral artery stenosis, lateralization of selec-

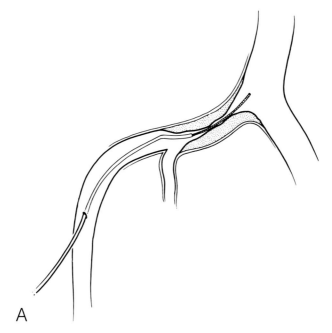

Fig. 25-1 (A) After angiographic identification of a treatable iliac stenosis, an angled tip catheter is used to carefully direct a guidewire through the lesion. (*Figure continues.*)

tive renal vein renins to the affected side supports a renal vascular etiology for the hypertension. Selective renins are somewhat imprecise, however, and failure to lateralize does not exclude a renovascular component.

In patients with fibromuscular disease and stenosis of the main renal artery or accessible lesions of segmental renal arteries without aneurysmal dilatation, angioplasty is the treatment of choice. Stenosis is more commonly due to atherosclerotic disease. The ideal lesion for angioplasty is a focal concentric stenosis of the main renal artery that does not involve the renal artery ostium and is not associated with severe aortic disease. Ostial renal artery lesions may be technicaly amenable to dilatation, but the likelihood of clinical benefit is less than for main renal artery lesions. Although preservation of renal function may be an indication for angioplasty in patients with renal insufficiency and bilateral renal artery stenosis, it has been less successful. Stenosis in a transplant renal artery may also be amenable to balloon angioplasty, with clinical benefits similar to those of surgical reconstruction and a lower risk of graft loss.

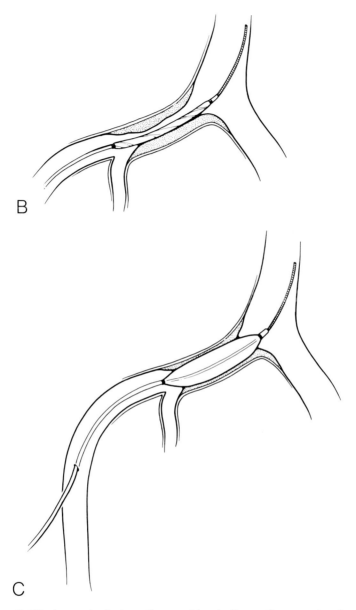

Fig. 25-1 (*Continued*) **(B)** An angioplasty catheter with a balloon of appropriate length and outer diameter is selected on the basis of the diagnostic angiogram. The balloon is positioned across the stenosis with the use of the radiopaque markers, which indicate the proximal and distal extent of the balloon. **(C)** The angioplasty balloon should inflate to its full diameter with no evidence of a waist. The presence of a waist may indicate a residual stenosis and suggests the need for a larger balloon.

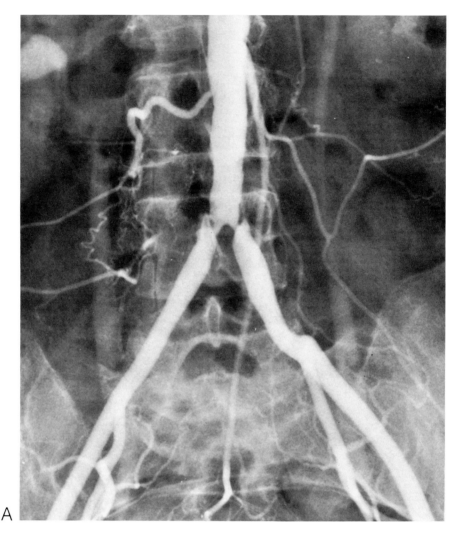

Fig. 25-2 (A) Diagnostic angiography performed for evaluation of bilateral lower extremity claudication reveals a tight stenosis at the origin of each common iliac artery. (*Figure continues.*)

Risks: Abdominal aortography, with the attendant risk of arterial entry and contrast material reaction, is usually performed prior to angioplasty. Renal artery spasm with occlusion, arterial dissection with resultant thrombosis, and, rarely, arterial rupture are risks specific to the performance of angioplasty.

Technique: In addition to the usual preangiographic evaluation and preparation, vascular surgical consultation should be obtained to assure the availability of emergency backup, should acute renal arterial occlusion or rupture occur during angioplasty. In patients with

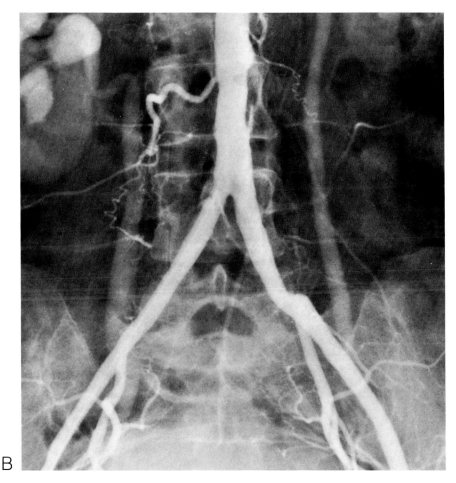

B

Fig. 25-2 (*Continued*). **(B)** Angiography following simultaneous angioplasty using a "double balloon" technique reveals wide patency of the vessels. The patient was without symptoms at a 3-year follow-up.

stenosis as a result of fibromuscular disease, nifedipine (10 mg) given orally the evening before the procedure may reduce the risk of renal artery spasm.

Angioplasty of the native renal arteries can usually be performed from the retrograde femoral artery approach. Transbrachial access may be required in rare instances because of a very steep caudal renal artery course. The transbrachial approach is usually avoided because of the risk of puncture site complications, especially in hypertensive patients who will be given heparin during the procedure, and in whom a sheath measuring 6 Fr or larger will be introduced.

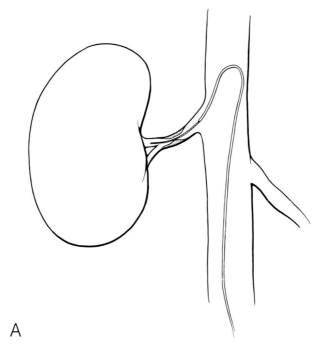

A

Fig. 25-3. (A) After documentation of a treatable renal artery lesion at diagnostic angiography, a reversed curve catheter is re-formed in the descending thoracic aorta. The catheter is withdrawn to engage the renal artery orfice, and a Bentson or other floppy tipped guidewire is carefully advanced through the stenosis. (*Figure continues.*)

After vascular access is established in a patient who has not previously undergone diagnostic aortography, a 4 to 5 Fr pigtail catheter is inserted over a standard J guidewire and positioned for abdominal aortography to evaluate the proximal renal arteries. Placing the patient in a slight right posterior oblique position may optimize evaluation of the renal artery origins. After catheter introduction, a heparin bolus (5,000 IU) is injected.

On the basis of the aortographic study, balloon size is determined by measuring the normal luminal diameter of the renal artery without correction for magnification to assure slight vessel overdilation, which is necessary for successful angioplasty. Measurements should not be made at sites of post-stenotic dilatation. A 5 Fr balloon angioplasty catheter with appropriate balloon diameter and a short catheter tip beyond the balloon minimizes vessel trauma. Following balloon selection, the pigtail catheter is removed over a guidewire, and a vascular introducer sheath is placed at the arterial entry site. A 6 Fr sheath is required for insertion of a balloon catheter with a 5 Fr shaft, and a 7 Fr sheath will accommodate both a 4 Fr pigtail and 0.035-in. guidewire (see

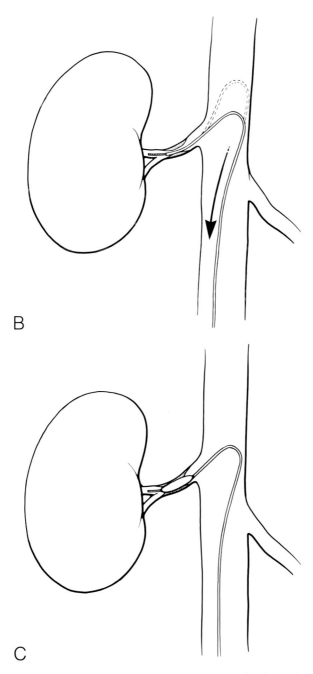

Fig. 25-3 (*Continued*) **(B)** After guidewire traversal of the stenosis, the catheter is advanced through the lesion by withdrawal of the catheter shaft at the skin entry site. With the tip of the catheter beyond the stenosis, the floppy guidewire is removed, the catheter position is confirmed with contrast material injection, and antispasmodics and anticoagulants are given. An exchange guidewire is then inserted, and the selective catheter removed. **(C)** An angioplasty catheter with a balloon of appropriate outer diameter and length is inserted over the guidewire and positioned across the stenosis. Inflation of the balloon to its full diameter should reveal no waist.

below). A catheter for selective renal artery entry and lesion traversal is then inserted over the guidewire. A Rösch left gastric or similar reversed curve catheter is used. Less commonly, an RC1 configuration is used. The reversed curve catheter is chosen to facilitate traversal of a tight stenosis and to allow catheterization of a downward slanting renal artery. The catheter curve is reformed in the descending aorta and retracted over a floppy-tipped J guidewire to the level of the renal arteries. The guidewire is removed and the catheter tip is carefully engaged in the renal artery orifice.

Catheter position is confirmed by careful hand-injection of contrast material. A Bentson guidewire is then advanced through the stenosis. For more difficult lesions, a steerable guidewire such as the TAD wire may be necessary. Following guidewire traversal, the catheter is advanced through the lesion. The guidewire is removed, the catheter flushed, and pressure is measured. Contrast material is injected to confirm that the catheter tip is in an intraarterial position distal to the stenotic lesion. A guidewire of sufficient length to maintain a position across the stenosis and allow exchange of the selective catheter for the balloon catheter is then inserted (180-cm Rosen or Moses wire, Cook, Bloomington, IN). The selective catheter is exchanged for the preselected balloon catheter. The balloon is positioned across the stenotic lesion with guidance from the control arteriogram, bony landmarks, or digital roadmapping. The balloon is inflated with a handle and in-line pressure gauge with dilute contrast material under constant fluoroscopic observation and with constant monitoring of balloon pressure. The patient is asked to note back pain or any discomfort associated with balloon inflation. A balloon waist is often observed as the stenosis is encountered. With further inflation, the waist should dissipate and the balloon contour should appear smooth. At this point, additional balloon pressure is not necessary (Fig. 25-3).

The balloon is left inflated for 45 s and then deflated to allow renal perfusion. An intraarterial injection of nitroglycerin (100 to 200 μg) is appropriate immediately before and after dilatation to combat renal arterial spasm. The balloon is reinflated at least once to confirm that the waist is no longer present. The balloon is completely deflated and then advanced slightly beyond the lesion, the guidewire is removed, and the balloon catheter is flushed. Contrast material is injected by hand to confirm antegrade renal arterial blood flow, and a pressure measurement is obtained.

If a 7 Fr or larger vascular introducer sheath has been employed to maintain access to the femoral artery, the balloon catheter can be removed over a 0.035-in. guidewire that is left in place across

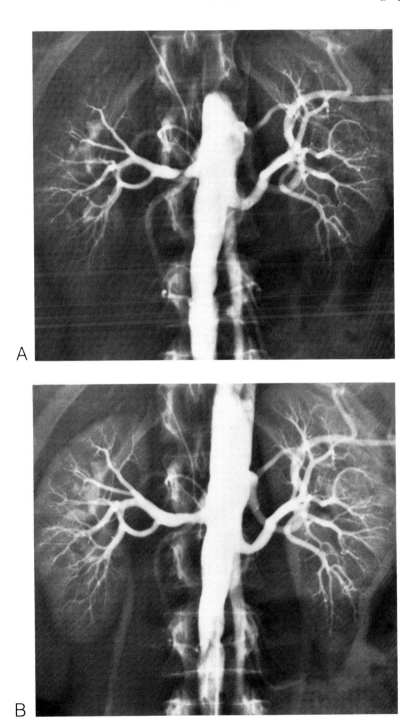

Fig. 25-4. (A) Diagnostic aortography in a patient with hypertension reveals an eccentric stenosis in the proximal main right renal artery, typical of atherosclerotic narrowing. **(B)** Aortography following balloon dilatation of the right renal artery reveals marked improvement in the luminal diameter. The patient became normotensive without medication within 48 h after the procedure.

the dilated renal artery lesion. A 4 Fr pigtail catheter can be inserted through the sheath adjacent to the wire for performance of postdilatation aortography. If review of the postdilatation films reveals a satisfactory angiographic result without evidence of complication (vessel occlusion, rupture), the pigtail catheter is removed and the selective endhole catheter repositioned across the exchange wire into the distal renal artery. Pressure can be measured distal to the lesion. The catheter is then retracted over a Bentson guidewire to prevent trauma to the freshly dilated lesion, and aortic pressure is measured for comparison. If at this point the result is satisfactory the catheter and introducer sheath are removed, and manual compression is applied at the puncture site.

Postprocedural Care: In addition to the usual postangiographic procedure orders, vital signs, particularly the pulse, blood pressure, and urinary output, must be monitored closely during the next 24 h. After successful renal angioplasty, antihypertensive therapy may require adjustment to avoid hypotension. In patients undergoing angioplasty to salvage renal function, diuretic response may be significant. Careful monitoring is necessary to avoid fluid and electrolyte depletion. Nearly all renal artery angioplasty patients receive chronic low-dose aspirin therapy to prevent platelet aggregation.

Results: In patients with fibromuscular disease, the technical success of balloon angioplasty is approximately 90% with a 93% rate of clinical benefit (58% cure rate and 35% improvement in hypertension control). For atherosclerotic disease, technical success rates are similar (Fig. 25-4); however, only about 70% of patients benefit clinically (29% cure rate and 41% improvement in hypertension control). Angioplasty of transplant renal artery stenosis carries a technical success rate greater than 80% with a significantly lower risk of graft loss than with surgical repair. Although restenosis has been reported in up to 20% of patients after transplant renal artery angioplasty, repeat dilatation in such cases is usually possible.

SUGGESTED READINGS

Becker GJ, Katzen BT, Dake MD: Noncoronary angioplasty. Radiology 170:921, 1989

Gardiner GA Jr, Meyerovitz MF, Stokes KR et al: Complications of transluminal angioplasty. Radiology 159:201, 1986

Katzen BT: Percutaneous transluminal angioplasty for arterial disease of the lower extremities. AJR 142:23, 1984

Martin LG, Casarella WJ, Gaylord GM: Azotemia caused by renal artery stenosis: treatment by percutaneous angioplasty. AJR 150:839, 1988

Raynaud A, Bedrossian J, Remy P et al: Percutaneous transluminal angioplasty of renal transplant arterial stenoses. AJR 146:853, 1986

Schwarten DE: Aortic, iliac, and peripheral arterial angioplasty. In Castaneda-Zuniga WR, Tadavarthy SM (eds): Interventional Radiology. Williams & Wilkins, Baltimore, 1992

Tegtmeyer CJ, Sos TA: Techniques of renal angioplasty. Radiology 161:577, 1986

26

Inferior Vena Cava Filters

Mark A. Yap
Ray Dyer

Indications: Requests for placement of inferior vena cava filters may occur in a variety of clinical situations, which include the following.

1. Documented pulmonary thromboembolism or deep venous thrombosis with a contraindication to anticoagulation (recent major surgery, bleeding peptic ulcer, intracranial hemorrhage).
2. Documented recurrent pulmonary thromboembolism in patients adequately treated with anticoagulants.
3. Pulmonary thromboembolism or deep venous thrombosis with complications of anticoagulation therapy (gastrointestinal bleeding, retroperitoneal hematoma, intracranial hemorrhage).
4. Chronic pulmonary hypertension secondary to recurrent pulmonary thromboembolism.
5. Septic pulmonary thromboembolism.
6. Postsurgical status after pulmonary embolectomy.
7. Prophylactic placement in patients with deep venous thrombosis who require major surgery or in patients at risk for pulmonary thromboembolism because of their condition (pelvic fractures).
8. Recurrent pulmonary thromboemblism in the elderly.

Risks: Placement of an inferior vena cava filter is preceded by venous cannulation and performance of inferior venacavography with the associated risks. Because large (up to 14 Fr) introduction sheaths must be inserted, the risk of bleeding and venous injury at the puncture site is greater, as is the potential for venous thrombosis following catheter removal. Preexisting thrombus in the inferior vena cava may be dislodged during inferior venacavography or filter placement. Because large-bore introducer sheaths are used, there is a risk of introducing air into the venous system during filter placement. The filter itself may be placed incorrectly, with a reduction in filtration efficiency. The filter may also perforate the vena cava wall, producing retroperitoneal hemorrhage. Filter migration may also occur, or recurrent pulmonary thromboembolism may recur despite appropriate filter placement. Inferior vena cava thrombosis is also reported following vena cava filter placement.

Technique: In patients referred for vena cava filter placement, there should be documented evidence of pulmonary thromboembolism, deep venous thrombosis, or other firm indications. Inferior venacavography should be performed before filter placement (see Ch. 20). It is helpful to have a ruler or grid in place beneath the patient and parallel to the inferior vena cava so that measurements of the caval diameter can be made with correction for radiographic magnification. Inferior venacavography can be performed with the catheter utilized for pulmonary angiography. The inferior vena cava filter is ideally placed below the inflow of the renal veins to prevent involvement with thrombosis that may occur in association with filter placement. Caval thrombus or anatomic abnormality that might alter standard filter placement should be noted. Three filters are widely available for percutaneous insertion. The femoral venous route is favored because of ease of insertion and familiarity to most operators. A jugular route can be used with appropriate equipment.

Greenfield Filter

The stainless steel Greenfield filter (GF) (Medi-tech, Watertown, MA) has the longest history of use. This filter is introduced into the vascular system by means of a 24 Fr carrier capsule. Insertion requires a venous cutdown, or dilatation of the venotomy site with a balloon dilatation catheter and large dilator sheath system. The newer titanium GF can be inserted through a 14 Fr sheath and can be placed with inferior vena cava diameters up to 28 mm. A right femoral venous approach is favored (Fig. 26-1).

Insertion Technique:
1. Following inferior venacavography, a 0.038-in. guidewire is placed in the inferior vena cava above the inflow of the renal veins.

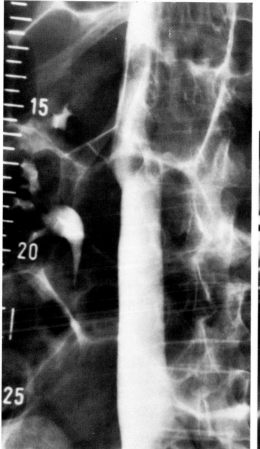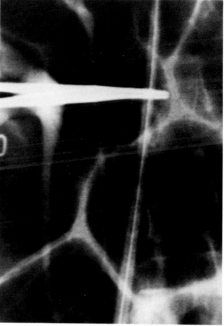

A   B

Fig. 26-1. (A) An inferior venacavogram with adjacent ruler is performed prior to filter placement. Renal vein inflow is seen between the 15 and 20 levels. **(B)** A point below which the GF may be deployed is marked with a hemostat and the dilator sheath unit is advanced into the cava. (*Figure continues.*)

2. The skin incision site is widened to 3 to 4 mm.
3. The dilator sheath unit for insertion of the filter is introduced, with the tip just above the level of the lowest renal vein.
4. The inner dilator and guidewire are withdrawn, and the sheath hub is occluded with the thumb.
5. The sheath is flushed with heparinized saline using the adaptor provided.
6. The introducer catheter with the preloaded titanium GF capsule is inserted into the sheath.
7. Under fluoroscopic control, the filter capsule is positioned at the release site.

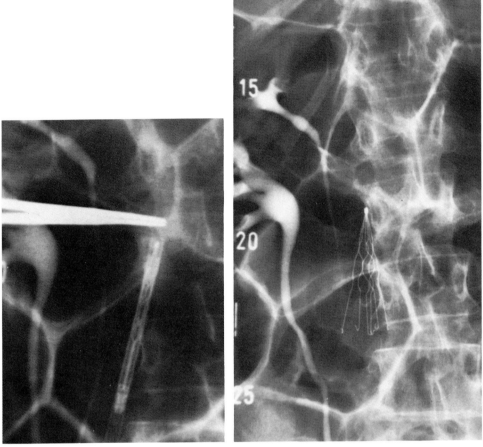

Fig. 26-1. (*Continued*). **(C)** The introducer catheter with the preloaded GF capsule is advanced through the sheath to the delivery position. **(D)** After deployment, a final film is obtained to document filter position.

8. The sheath is then retracted onto the introducer catheter at the skin, to completely uncover the preloaded filter capsule.
9. The safety handle is then used to uncover the filter and allow its discharge.
10. After placement, a follow-up abdominal radiograph is obtained to document the filter position. Inferior venacavography may be performed through the sheath by reattachment of the flush adaptor to the sheath hub prior to its removal.

Bird's Nest Filter

The bird's nest filter (BNF) (Cook, Bloomington, IN) was the first available with a small-bore (12 Fr) carrier. Placement is possible with inferior vena cava diameters up to 40 mm (Fig. 26-2).

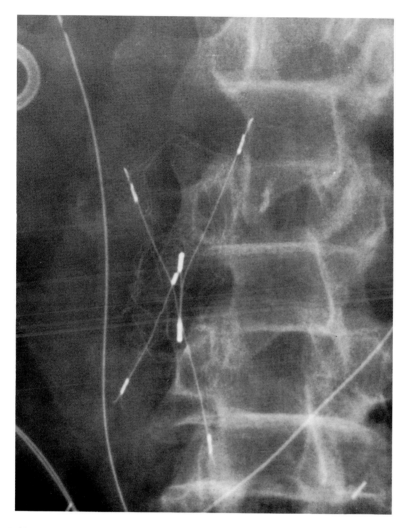

Fig. 26-2. A film after delivery of a BNF shows overlap of the distal and proximal junction points. The nest of interwoven wires is barely visible.

Insertion Technique:

1. Following inferior venacavography, a 0.038-in. guidewire is placed in the inferior vena cava above the inflow of the renal veins.
2. The venotomy site is enlarged to 3 to 4 mm.
3. The filter introducer sheath is inserted until the hub reaches the skin. The filter catheter is filled with contrast material, and after removal of the guidewire and inner dilator, the filter catheter is introduced into the sheath and secured with the Luer rock. The catheter tip extends 1.5 cm beyond the introducer sheath. This tip is positioned at the discharge point of the distal hooks of the BNF.

4. The hemostatic valve is then loosened.
5. The pusher wire is held stationary and the sheath–catheter assembly is withdrawn over the wire to the premarked line. This maneuver discharges the distal anchoring hooks. The entire assembly is then advanced 1 to 3 mm to secure the distal anchoring hooks into the inferior vena cava wall.
6. The sheath–catheter assembly is then withdrawn an additional 1 to 3 cm over the pusher wire.
7. The wire guide pusher assembly is then advanced until the junction point of the proximal hook wires is seen at the catheter tip. This procedure creates the "nest" of redundant wires in the vessel lumen.
8. The entire assembly is then advanced so that the junction points of the distal and proximal anchoring hooks are in close proximity, or overlap by 2 to 3 cm, ensuring adequate formation of the filter "nest."
9. The sheath–catheter assembly is then withdrawn over the wire to the right angle bend while the pusher wire is held steady. This maneuver releases the proximal anchoring hooks.
10. The hooks are then secured into the vena cava wall with a slight "to-and-fro" motion.
11. The right angle handle of the wire guide pusher is then turned 10 to 15 times *counterclockwise* to disengage it from the filter. The empty filter catheter is then removed, and a follow-up abdominal film or repeat venacavogram can be obtained through the introducer sheath.

Vena-Tech Filter

The Vena-Tech filter (Vena-Tech, Brookline, MA) can be introduced through a 12 Fr sheath and can be placed with inferior vena cava diameters up to 28 mm. A right femoral venous approach is favored (Fig. 26-3).

Insertion Technique:
1. Following inferior venacavography, a 0.038-in. guidewire is placed with the tip above the inflow of the renal veins.
2. The venotomy site is enlarged to 3 to 4 mm.
3. The syringe containing the preloaded filter is flushed with heparinized saline. After the dilator sheath insertion set is introduced, the radiopaque marker of the dilator is placed at the anticipated position of the upper level of the filter when deployed. The marker collar on the sheath external to the patient is then seated snugly at the skin to stabilize the sheath position.
4. The inner dilator with the radiopaque marker is removed.

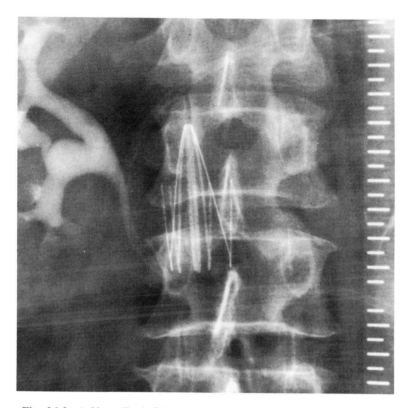

Fig. 26-3. A Vena-Tech filter is in appropriate position after delivery.

5. The preflushed syringe containing the filter is attached to the sheath, and the filter is injected into it.
6. The filter is advanced into the introducer sheath with the pusher catheter to the premarked line to position the filter for deployment.
7. The filter is delivered by stabilizing the pusher catheter and pulling the outer sheath back over the pusher in a fast, smooth motion.
8. The pusher catheter is withdrawn. An abdominal film is obtained, and repeat inferior venacavography may be performed through the placement sheath prior to its removal.

SUGGESTED READINGS

Grassi CJ: Inferior vena caval filters: analysis of five currently available devices. AJR 156:813, 1991

Greenfield LJ, Cho KJ, Pais SO, Van Aman M: Preliminary clinical experience with the titanium Greenfield vena caval filter. Arch Surg 124:657, 1989

Greenfield LF, Cho KJ, Proctor M et al: Results of a multicenter study of the modified hook–titanium Greenfield filter. J Vasc Surg 14:253, 1991

Mewissen MW, Erickson SJ, Foley WD et al: Thrombosis at venous insertion sites after inferior vena caval filter placement. Radiology 173:155, 1989

Murphy TP, Dorfman GS, Yedlicka JW et al: LGM vena cava filter: objective evaluation of early results. J Vasc Intervent Radiol 2:107, 1991

Ricco JB, Crochet D, Sebilotte P et al: Percutaneous transvenous caval interruption with the "LGM" filter: early results of a multicenter trial. Ann Vasc Surg 3:242, 1988

Roehm JOF Jr, Gianturco C, Barth MH: The bird's nest inferior vena caval filter. Semin Intervent Radiol 3:205, 1986

Roehm JOF Jr, Johnsrude IS, Barth MH, Gianturco C: The bird's nest inferior vena cava filter: progress report. Radiology 168:745, 1988

27

Fibrinolytic Therapy

Augustin G. Formanek

Definition: Clinically effective fibrinolytic therapy implies the rapid dissolution of preformed thrombi with preservation of organ function in arterial occlusion, or valvular competence in venous occlusion. Selective intraarterial infusion of lytic agents as an alternative method to intravenous application achieves maximal thrombolysis with minimal systemic lytic effects.

Indications: Fibrinolytic therapy with direct application of therapeutic agents into the site of blockage is the initial method of choice to recanalize vessels occluded by blood clots. Arterial occlusions are most often the result of atherosclerotic disease. The site of occlusion may be within the native artery or in surgically inserted bypass grafts. Any patient who tolerates an acute occlusion (less than 10 days) is a good candidate for fibrinolytic therapy. A successful outcome is less often achieved with chronic thrombotic occlusions.

Mechanism: To induce thrombolysis in occlusive vascular disease, a plasminogen activator in the form of streptokinase, human urokinase, or tissue plasminogen activator is administered directly into the occluding blood clot. The plasminogen activators bind avidly to fibrin (the essential component of the blood clot), and circulating plasminogen in turn binds to the formed plasminogen activator–fibrin complex. This complex is converted into plasmin, a trypsin-like protein that is capable of hydrolyzing fibrin.

Streptokinase, a catabolic by-product of group C-beta-hemolytic *Streptococci*, is an *indirect* activator. It first combines with plasminogen to form a plasminogen–streptokinase complex, which then converts uncomplexed plasminogen to plasmin. Streptokinase is a foreign protein and therefore an antigen.

Urokinase, isolated from human urine, is a *direct* activator. It initiates fibrinolysis without forming an activator complex and has a rapid onset of action. It is not antigenic.

Tissue plasminogen activator is not commonly used for treatment of peripheral vascular occlusive disease.

Plasmin is a nonspecific proteolytic enzyme that, in addition to fibrin, digests clotting factors I (fibrinogen), II (prothrombin), V (proaccelerin), and VII (antihemophilic factor). Therefore, its activation may result in a systemic lytic state causing lysis of all fresh thrombi, proteolytic destruction of the noted clotting factors, and increase in fibrin degradation products.

Risks: In addition to contrast material reaction or bleeding at the site of catheter entry, risks related to fibrinolytic therapy include bleeding at a remote site, peripheral embolization caused by fragmentation of lysed clots, or dislodgement of central thrombi, especially from an intracardiac location. These risks are related to local or systemic fibrinolytic effects. However, these events are not caused by biochemical changes in the coagulation factors, but by disintegration of existing thrombotic plugs. Therefore, careful selection of patients decreases the rate of major complications.

Absolute contraindications for fibrinolytic therapy are active internal bleeding, recent cerebrovascular accidents, known intracranial tumor, or neurosurgical interventions within 2 months. Relative contraindications are conditions requiring formation of hemostatic plugs within 10 days of initiation of therapy. These conditions include major surgery, a postpartum state, or recent serious trauma. Practically, coagulability decreases after a short period of therapy in all patients.

Laboratory monitoring of thrombin, fibrinogen, and its degradation products is the best reflection of the status of the fibrinolytic system, but does not ensure prevention of hemorrhagic complications because of the poor correlation between laboratory derangement of clotting factors and a tendency for bleeding. The value of laboratory tests is to assure that a fibrinolytic state is achieved and to avoid profound hypofibrinogenemia (<50 mg). Major hemorrhagic events occur in 6% of treated patients, most commonly at the site of infusion catheter entry. Such occurrences may require discontinuation of therapy or blood transfusions. If bleeding occurs at a site other than that of catheter entry, surgical evacuation of the hematoma is often necessary. Minor bleeding at the catheter entry site can often be controlled by application of local pressure or insertion of a larger bore catheter.

***Choice of
Thrombolytic
Agent:***
In general, urokinase is preferred to streptokinase for the following reasons.

1. Urokinase is not an antigen. Patients with elevated streptokinase antibody titer from previous *Streptococcus* infection have a decreased rate of success with low-dose streptokinase infusion therapy.
2. Complete clot lysis with urokinase occurs in 75% to 80% of patients, whereas lysis with streptokinase is seen in only 45% to 60%.
3. The average duration of infusion therapy is shorter with urokinase (18 h) than with streptokinase (41 h). The higher cost of urokinase is often offset by the shorter duration of infusion therapy.

Technique:
The procedure is initiated under fluoroscopic control. A baseline diagnostic arteriogram is required for planning of the therapeutic approach and appraisal of progress and end result. Because the puncture site for positioning the infusion catheter should be as close as possible to the site of occlusion (to minimize the propensity for clot formation around the catheter), diagnostic angiography is often performed from a contralateral or upper extremity approach. The therapeutic catheter is then introduced from the ipsilateral side, in antegrade fashion. A one-wall arterial puncture technique is preferable because it decreases the likelihood of local bleeding complications. To avoid stasis in the vessel proximal to the occlusion, the smallest catheter possible (3 to 4 Fr straight catheter with multiple side holes) is introduced over a suitable guidewire and embedded within the proximal portion of the occluding clot. As a result, the fibrinolytic agent is delivered directly into the thrombus. Prior to this maneuver, an attempt should be made to traverse the entire clot with a guidewire (Bentson, Glidewire). This helps the lytic agent penetrate the clot more efficiently and mechanically disrupts the clot. The ease with which the guidewire can be advanced through the clot is a simple predictor of therapeutic outcome. Easy passage indicates a soft, unorganized clot with a high likelihood of complete lysis.

Urokinase infusion is begun at a dose rate of 4,000 IU/min (urokinase preparation: 500,000 IU is diluted in 200 cc of normal saline, yielding 2,500 IU/cc. This preparation is infused at a rate of 96 cc/h with an appropriate pump). A hand-injected bolus of 10,000 IU (4 cc of the infusion solution) may be delivered prior to the start of continuous infusion.

After 2 to 4 h, angiography is repeated to assure that the catheter position is unchanged, to assess whether fibrinolysis has been achieved, and to adjust catheter position more distally into the residual clot to improve therapeutic efficiency and shorten the duration of infusion. Depending on the extent of initial lysis, infusion is continued either at full strength (no or minimal lysis) for another 3 to 4 h. If considerable lysis has occurred, the dose is reduced to 1,000 to 2,000 IU/min for an additional 6 to 8 h. If after 8 h of therapy no signs of lysis can be seen and laboratory studies show a systemic lytic effect, therapy is discontinued. Otherwise, the infusion rate of 1,000 IU/min is continued and the results checked with fluoroscopy every 8 h. Catheter repositioning into the residual clot is repeated until complete recanalization of the vessel is achieved (Fig. 27-1).

Small residual clots often remain adherent to the vessel wall. In such cases, the therapeutic catheter is pulled back to the original level and infusion with 1,000 IU/min is continued. In approximately half of the treated patients distal embolization of small clot fragments occurs; however, only rarely do they cause symptoms. If symptoms do result, the catheter is advanced distally, if possible, into the embolized artery, and infusion is continued at 2,000 IU/min until dissolution occurs.

Therapy is terminated when no residual clots are seen. Angiography at this time often reveals the primary cause of thrombosis, either significant stenosis from atherosclerotic disease or stenosis at the site of bypass graft anastomosis. To prevent rethrombosis, the stenotic lesion should be treated either with percutaneous transluminal angioplasty or with surgical revision. Percutaneous angioplasty can be performed immediately because of the short half-life of plasminogen activators (10 to 12 min).

There is debate concerning concomitant infusion of heparin and fibrinolytic agents to prevent pericatheter thrombus formation during therapy. Advocates of heparin administration suggest that it prevents thrombus formation. The alternate view states that a systemic lytic condition produces decreased coagulability and the addition of heparin serves only to increase the tendency for bleeding complications. If heparin is administered, intravenous infusion of 1,000 IU/h can be used, or direct intraarterial delivery can be performed via the side arm of a 5 Fr introducer sheath, through which the therapeutic catheter is placed. The partial thromboplastin time should be maintained at a level 2.5 to 3 times the normal value.

If streptokinase is used for fibrinolysis, the usual starting dose is 5,000 to 10,000 IU/h. Tapering of the infusion rate depends on the progression of fibrinolysis.

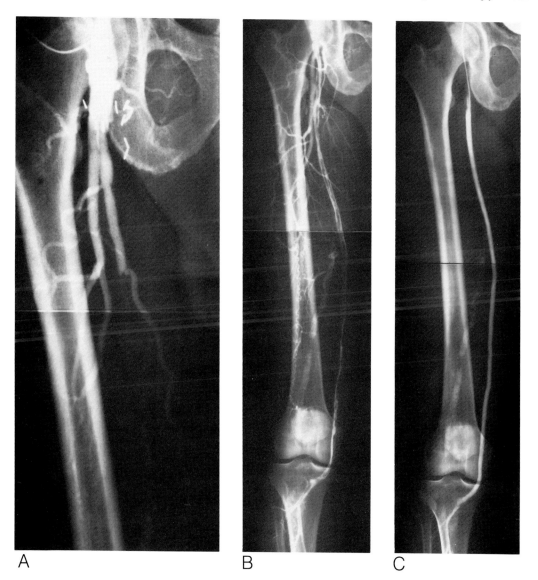

A   B   C

Fig. 27-1. **(A)** Arteriography was performed in this patient who developed acute lower limb ischemia 6 months after femoral–popliteal bypass grafting. Surgical clips mark the proximal anastamotic site, but the graft is occluded, as is the superficial femoral artery. **(B)** Following antegrade puncture of the right common femoral artery, the graft was successfully entered and a ''tunnel'' created in the occluding clot with a guidewire. Some flow is now seen in the popliteal artery below the knee. **(C)** Repeat arteriography after 14 h of urokinase infusion at a rate of 2,000 IU/min shows a patent graft. Note the densely calcified superficial femoral and popliteal artery lateral to the graft.

The long-term clinical results of fibrinolytic therapy are best in thrombotic occlusions of native lower extremity vessels, in which patency of the recanalized vessel is 81% after 2 yr. In occluded lower extremity bypass grafts, initial success is 69%, and overall graft patency at the end of 1 yr is about 60%. Attempts to salvage irreparably damaged tissue (ischemic necrosis) must be avoided because of the grave risk of compartment syndrome, which, if not relieved, can lead to myoglobinuria, oliguria, hyperkalemia, and even death.

Some Associated Considerations

1. Before initiation of fibrinolytic therapy, full consultation and cooperation among the referring physician, radiologist, and vascular surgeon should be assured.
2. Baseline laboratory levels of hemoglobin, hematocrit, thrombin, fibrinogen, and fibrin degradation products are obtained at the start of the infusion and every 8 to 12 h during the infusion.
3. To minimize bleeding complications, parenteral injections or additional arterial or venous punctures are avoided during therapy.
4. The indwelling catheter is secured in place with tape rather than sutures.
5. The puncture site for the infusion catheter should be accessible for good manual compression in the event local bleeding complications occur.
6. The patient should be monitored in a care setting with a high nurse to patient ratio.
7. The femoral and popliteal arteries are the most common sites for performance of fibrinolytic therapy. Because these are not considered high-flow vessels, anticoagulant therapy is indicated after successful fibrinolysis. Initial intravenous heparin infusion at 1,000 IU/h can be replaced after a few days with warfarin derivatives or platelet aggregation inhibitors.

SUGGESTED READINGS

Becker GJ, Holden RW (eds): Fibrinolysis. Semin Intervent Radiol 2:315, 1985

Durham JD, Geller SC, Abbott WM et al: Regional infusion of urokinase into occluded lower-extremity bypass grafts: long-term clinical results. Radiology 172:83, 1989

Katzen BT: Technique and results of ''low-dose'' infusion. Cardiovasc Intervent Radiol 11:S41, 1988

Lammer J, Pilger E, Neumayer K, Schreyer H: Intraarterial fibrinolysis: long-term results. Radiology 161:159, 1986

McNamara T: Technique and results of ''higher-dose'' infusion. Cardiovasc Intervent Radiol 11:S48, 1988

McNamara TO: Role of thrombolysis in peripheral arterial occlusion. Am J Med, 83 Suppl. 2A:6, 1987

Palaskas C, Totty WG, Gilula LA, Reinus WR: Complications of local intra-arterial fibrinolytic therapy. Semin Intervent Radiol 2:396, 1985

Saldinger E, Bookstein JJ: Mechanisms of fibrinolysis: native and exogenous systems, Semin Intervent Radiol 2:321, 1985

Sharma GVRK, Cella G, Parisi AF, Sasahara AA: Thrombolytic therapy. N Engl J Med 306:1268, 1982

van Breda A, Katzen BT, Deutsch AS: Urokinase versus streptokinase in local thrombolysis. Radiology 165:109, 1987

28

Therapeutic Embolization

Vincent J. D'Souza

Indications: Therapeutic vascular embolization may be indicated in a number of clinical situations. These include traumatic bleeding, especially in pelvic trauma (procedure of choice); gastrointestinal bleeding when pharmacologic methods of control have failed or when the patient is not a surgical candidate; arteriovenous communication, either traumatic (procedure of choice) or congenital; and ablation of kidneys in patients with hypertension and end-stage renal disease. For some tumors, such as hypervascular hepatomas, embolization with adjunctive chemotherapeutic agents may be used. Use of embolization for hypernephromas is controversial.

Materials: Agents used for embolization are divided into those that produce temporary occlusion and those that produce permanent occlusion.

Temporary:
Gelfoam (Upjohn, Kalamazoo, MI) is the easiest and most commonly used material, producing occlusion that lasts from days to weeks.

Permanent:
Gianturco steel coils (Cook, Bloomington, IN) are the easiest and most commonly used permanent occluding device. Absolute ethanol can be used but is somewhat more cumbersome. Bucrylate, often referred to as glue, polyvinyl alcohol (Ivalon, Interventional Therapeutics Corporation, San Francisco, CA) and detachable balloons are used in certain research locales, but are not widely available.

Risks: Migration of embolic materials to an undesirable location is a relatively serious complication depending on the type of embolic materials. For example, Gelfoam particles that are small enough

229

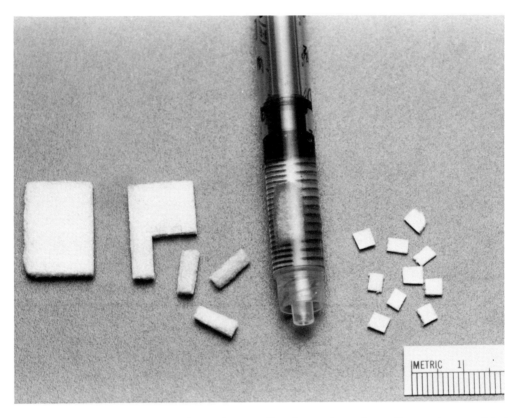

Fig. 28-1. A sheet of Gelfoam can be cut into small or large pieces depending on the vessel to be occluded. A syringe contains a single 2 × 10-mm piece prepared for injection.

to pass through an arteriovenous malformation can lodge in the lung. The same is true for small steel coils.

Reflux of steel coils or Gelfoam proximal to the catheter tip can occur during embolization once the blood flow slows substantially. Caution must be exercised once slowing of blood flow is seen at fluoroscopy. Bowel infarction has been attributed to the use of ethanol in renal ablation because of reflux into the inferior mesenteric artery. Also, permanent damage to the sacral nerve plexus is possible during embolization of pelvic arteriovenous malformations.

Catheterization: Catheter selection for embolization depends on the source vessel to undergo occlusion. See the appropriate angiographic section for details.

Technique: After demonstrating a target vessel for occlusion, selective or superselective catheterization is carried out. If temporary occlusion is required, Gelfoam is the material of choice because of its availability and the ease with which it can be injected.

Depending on the size of the vessel to be embolized, single or multiple pieces of Gelfoam as small as 2 to 3 mm are injected using a 3-cc syringe (Fig. 28-1). The pieces are mixed with dilute contrast material to allow monitoring during injection. Injection of any particulate matter is carried out in a slow, controlled manner under fluoroscopic observation to avoid reflux of embolic material. When blood flow in the vessel slows substantially in response to embolization, utmost care is necessary to avoid this complication.

Gelfoam is easily compressible and can be delivered through any catheter, including those with tapered tips. Occlusion lasts for days to weeks, after which the Gelfoam plug is recanalized. This temporary occlusion is ideal in the treatment of gastrointestinal or post-traumatic bleeding (Fig. 28-2).

Gianturco coils are made of stainless steel with Dacron fiber strands interwoven throughout the length of the coil. The appearance has been likened to that of a centipede or a pipe cleaner. Coils are available commercially in sizes based on the diameter of the coil wire (0.018 to 0.038 in.) and outside helix diameter (2 to 15 mm) preloaded in small cartridges (Fig. 28-3). These can be delivered through any catheter that will accept a compatible guidewire. The size of the coil chosen depends on the size of the vessel to be embolized. Too large a coil has a tendency to displace the catheter during delivery and may result in a coil protrusion into an undesirable location. Too small a coil may migrate beyond the desired occlusion site. Steel coils are ideal for occlusion of pelvic bleeding sites after disruption of internal iliac artery branches, arteriovenous malformation, or varicocele.

A combination of embolic materials is used when there is a need to occlude small vessels in addition to large feeding vessels, as in congenital arteriovenous malformations. Following catheterization of the source vessel, Gelfoam is used to occlude small vessels, and coils are used to occlude large feeding vessels. Pulmonary arteriovenous malformations tend to have a single arterial connection to a large pulmonary vein. Small particulate material such as Gelfoam maybe be carried into the systemic circulation through large arteriovenous communications.

Embolization at the small vessel level can be carried out with absolute ethanol. A common site of ethanol ablation is the kidney, where hypervascular tumors such as hypernephromas, or the entire vascular field in patients with hypertension and end-stage renal disease, may be ablated (Fig. 28-4). Absolute ethanol in divided doses with a total volume of 5 to 12 cc is injected very slowly into the main renal artery. This is done preferably after occluding the main renal artery with a balloon occlusion catheter

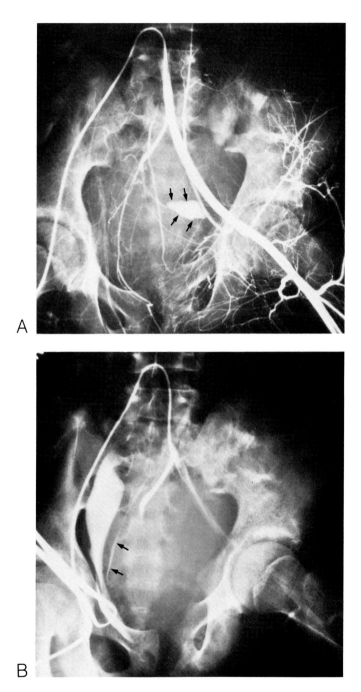

Fig. 28-2. (A) A left common iliac arteriogram performed for evaluation of continued blood loss after pelvic trauma from a motor vehicle accident reveals an area of brisk extravasation (*arrows*) from the left superior gluteal artery. **(B)** Gelfoam was used to embolize the bleeding site and repeat left internal iliac arteriography confirms successful occlusion. Note the deviation of the bladder and left ureter (*arrows*) caused by the large pelvic hematoma.

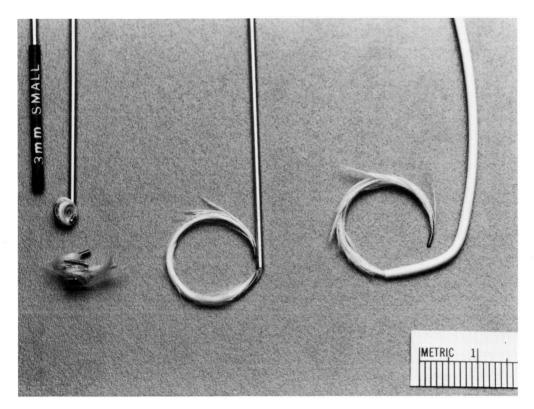

Fig. 28-3. A 0.038 in. × 3 mm × 3 cm coil has been extruded from its holder, and a second coil is partially extruded. A 0.038 in. × 15 mm × 5 cm coil is partially extruded from its holder, and a second coil is seen exiting a catheter. Note the interwoven fibers, which promote platelet aggregation.

to avoid reflux of ethanol and resultant nontarget injury. Ethanol has a tendency to gravitate into the origin of the inferior mesenteric or lumbar arteries. During ablation of arteriovenous malformations in the pelvis, permanent damage to the sacral neural plexus has been reported in some instances.

Polyvinyl alcohol (Ivalon), a material similar to that used in kitchen sponges, is a permanent occlusive material that causes little inflammatory reaction. This material expands when wet and has a high coefficient of friction, making it difficult to inject through a catheter. It is available in several sizes, including a powder with particles measuring 300 μ. Currently, this material is not generally available.

Other permanently occluding materials include detachable balloons and bucrylate. At present, these agents are available only on an investigational basis.

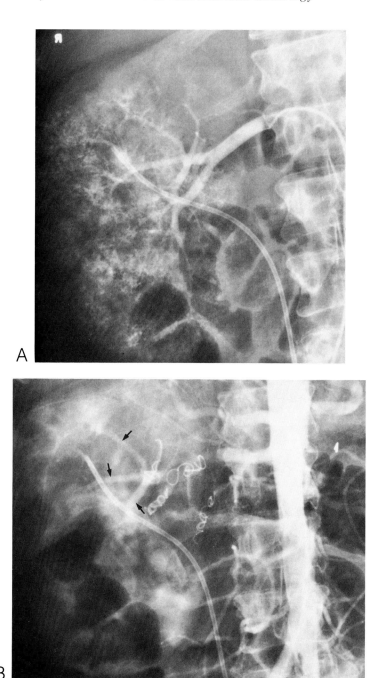

Fig. 28-4. (A) Renal arteriography in a patient with uncontrollable hematuria demonstrates a diffusely infiltrating hypervascular renal cell carcinoma in the right kidney. **(B)** Aortography after absolute ethanol injection and branch renal artery occlusion with steel coils shows complete renal artery thrombosis. Intravascular stagnation of contrast material distal to coils in the upper pole is seen (*arrows*).

SUGGESTED READINGS

Amplatz K, Coleman CC (eds): Therapeutic embolization of thorax and abdomen. Semin Intervent Radiol 1:95, 1984

Prochaska JM, Flye MW, Johnsrude IS: Left gastric artery embolization for control of gastric bleeding: a complication. Radiology 107:521, 1973

Reuter SR, Chuang VP, Bree RL: Selective arterial embolization for control of massive upper gastrointestinal bleeding. AJR 125:119, 1975

Sniderman KW, Franklin J Jr, Sos TA: Successful transcatheter Gelfoam embolization of a bleeding cecal vascular ectasia. AJR 131:157, 1978

Stanley RJ, Cubillo E: Nonsurgical treatment of arteriovenous malformations of the trunk and limb by transcatheter arterial embolization. Radiology 115:609, 1975

Tadavarthy SM, Moller JH, Amplatz K: Polyvinyl alcohol (Ivalon)—a new embolic material. AJR 125:609, 1975

Wallace S, Gianturco C, Anderson JH et al: Therapeutic vascular occlusion utilizing steel coil technique: clinical applications. AJR 127:381, 1976

White RI Jr, Kaufman SL, Barth KH et al: Therapeutic embolization with detachable silicone balloons: early clinical experience. JAMA 241:1257, 1979

White RI Jr, Strandberg JV, Gross GS, Barth KH: Therapeutic embolization with long-term occluding agents and their effects on embolized tissues. Radiology 125:677, 1977

Woodside J, Schwarz H, Bergreen P: Peripheral embolization complicating bilateral renal infarction with Gelfoam. AJR 126:1033, 1976

29

Percutaneous Biliary Intervention

William D. Routh

DIAGNOSTIC PERCUTANEOUS TRANSHEPATIC CHOLANGIOGRAPHY

Indications: Diagnostic percutaneous transhepatic cholangiography is performed for evaluation of known or suspected biliary pathology not adequately delineated by less invasive imaging techniques. This procedure is also performed as a preliminary step in percutaneous transhepatic biliary drainage.

Risks: Contrast material is used for opacification of the ducts, and because vascular beds are transgressed, there is a risk of contrast reaction. Bleeding, sepsis, bile leak with development of bile peritonitis, and pneumothorax are risks specifically associated with performance of the procedure.

Injection: An intermediate iodine concentration contrast material is used for ductal opacification (300 mg I/ml).

Filming: The biliary ductal system is usually filmed using 14 × 14-in. films and/or 105-mm spot films in anteroposterior and multiple oblique projections to define pathologic processes and to map the biliary system prior to drainage.

Technique: The coagulation status of the patient should be evaluated, and any abnormality should be corrected prior to beginning the procedure. In more urgent situations, such as cholangitis with sepsis in the context of obstruction, percutaneous transhepatic cholangiography and biliary drainage may have to be performed as attempts at correction of coagulopathy are ongoing.

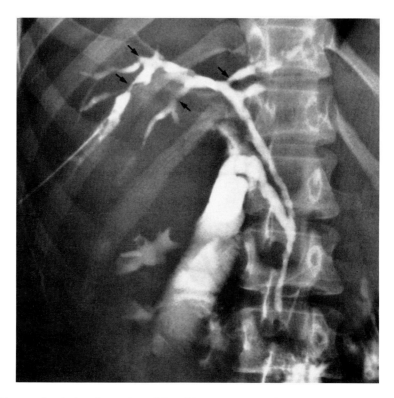

Fig. 29-1. Diagnostic cholangiography with a 22-gauge needle in a patient with jaundice reveals multiple intrahepatic bile duct strictures (arrows) consistent with a diagnosis of sclerosing cholangitis.

For patients without symptoms or signs of biliary tract infection, antibiotic prophylaxis with an intravenous broad-spectrum cephalosporin is begun immediately prior to the procedure. Patients with symptoms or signs of cholangitis may have already begun antibiotic therapy, and this is continued. If cholangiography reveals no evidence of biliary abnormality and the patient manifests no symptoms or signs of infection during the procedure, antibiotic therapy is discontinued. In patients with biliary obstruction, especially those in whom cholangiography has been a preliminary step to biliary drainage, antibiotic therapy is continued for 24 to 48 h or until the patient's clinical condition warrants discontinuation. Any available cross-sectional imaging studies and a preliminary radiograph of the upper abdomen are reviewed. A skin entry site is chosen in the right midaxillary line midway between the right costophrenic angle and the inferior edge of the liver as viewed fluoroscopically. The patient is asked to suspend respiration in midcycle during selection of the entry point. 1% lidocaine without epinephrine is infiltrated subcutaneously and along the anticipated needle track down to the river capsule, passing immediately cephalad to the rib to avoid injury to the intercostal vessel. A 2 to 3 mm incision is created and blunt dissection is performed with a hemostat. A 21- or 22-gauge diamond-tipped needle (Greene needle, Cook, Bloomington, IN) is introduced through the skin down to the liver capsule. The patient is instructed to suspend respiration. The needle is advanced in a single rapid, smooth motion under fluoroscopic guidance toward the central aspect of the right hepatic lobe. Care is taken to avoid the porta hepatis region because of the risk of injury to a central hepatic arterial branch. For opacification of an obstructed left ductal system, the needle can be passed more ventrally across the midline into the left lobe.

After a needle pass, the patient is allowed to breathe quietly. The needle stylet is removed, and contrast material is gently injected by hand as the needle is slowly retracted under fluoroscopic observation. Entry of the needle tip into a biliary radicle should produce characteristic slow flow away from the needle tip toward the liver hilus. If this is not observed on the first pass, the stylet is reintroduced and the needle is redirected for subsequent needle passes. To minimize the risk of bleeding and bile leakage, care is taken to avoid retraction of the needle tip through the liver capsule.

Once a stable intraductal needle tip position is achieved, contrast material is injected for cholangiographic filming (Fig. 29-1). If fluoroscopic observation reveals definite biliary pathology necessitating biliary drainage, care should be taken to prevent overdistention of the ducts, which may produce sepsis.

During attempted bile duct cannulation, excessive parenchymal staining by extravasated contrast material should be avoided because it may compromise the diagnostic quality of the examination.

PERCUTANEOUS TRANSHEPATIC BILIARY DRAINAGE

Indications: Indications for percutaneous transhepatic biliary drainage include palliative decompression of malignant biliary obstruction; acute decompression in patients with cholangitis and biliary obstruction; access for endoluminal biliary manipulations including stricture dilation, stone extraction, endoprosthesis placement, endoluminal irradiation, diagnostic cholangioscopy, or endoluminal biopsy; and nonoperative management of biliary fistulas.

Risks: The risks of percutaneous transhepatic biliary drainage are similar to those of diagnostic percutaneous transhepatic cholangiography and include contrast reaction, bleeding, sepsis, bile peritonitis, pneumothorax, or biliary–pleural fistula. Long-term complications of indwelling biliary drainage catheters include pericatheter bile leakage, recurrent jaundice, or cholangitis, all typically resulting from catheter occlusion. Skin irritation at the catheter entry site is to be expected. Significant pericatheter soft tissue infection is uncommon. Delayed hemorrhage or infected biloma can occur.

Technique: The presence of ascites should be considered a relative contraindication to biliary drainage because of the likelihood of persistent pericatheter leakage of ascitic fluid. Diffuse hepatic metastases are also a relative contraindication. It is unlikely that a biliary drainage catheter will palliate jaundice in such cases, due to the multifocality of the obstructing metastases. Diagnostic cholangiography is performed for mapping of the biliary ductal system before the performance of the drainage procedure. For high-grade biliary obstruction, care is taken to avoid overdistention of the bile ducts during contrast injection to decrease the risk of sepsis.

For right-sided biliary drainage, a relatively peripheral intrahepatic duct in the right lobe of the liver should be entered to provide sufficient purchase in the biliary tree to allow catheter and guidewire negotiation through the obstructing lesion(s) into the duodenum. To reduce the risk of hemorrhage, entry into central ducts (near the porta hepatis) should be avoided. After a suitable duct has been selected for entry, the site is prepared as outlined in the percutaneous transhepatic cholangiography section. A "single stick" entry system (Accustik, Medi-tech, Watertown, MA) is used. This system employs a 21-gauge diamond-tipped needle with an 0.018-in. monofilament stainless steel platinum-tipped guidewire and coaxial 4 and 6 Fr tapered dilators with a metal stiffening cannula.

The needle is passed into the liver and directed toward the opacified duct. Complex craniocaudal–oblique angulated fluoroscopy can aid in determination of the relationship of the needle tip to the opacified duct. When the needle contacts the duct, the wall can usually be seen to indent, and with further advancement the needle will enter or traverse the duct lumen. The platinum-tipped guidewire is advanced into the duct lumen. Advancement may be facilitated by placing a small amount of angulation in the tip of the guidewire prior to its introduction. The guidewire is advanced until all of the platinum tip and a portion of the stiffer stainless steel mandrel has entered the duct. The coaxial dilator system with the stiffening cannula is then advanced over the guidewire into the biliary tree. To avoid bile duct injury, care is taken not to advance the metallic stiffening cannula too far into the biliary system. Kinking of the platinum wire should also be avoided, as a kinked wire can separate upon withdrawal of the bent area through the metallic cannula or dilator.

When a stable intraductal position is established with the entry dilators, the stiffening cannula and smaller inner dilator are removed, leaving only the platinum-tipped wire in place as a "safety" guidewire through the larger outer dilator. A 0.038-in. working wire is inserted. The strictured area may require negotiation as outlined for vascular stenoses. Once the stricture is traversed and a catheter passed distally to the stricture, a heavy-duty guidewire (Lunderquist–Ring guidewire, heavy-duty floppy or 3-mm J guidewire, Lunderquist exchange guidewire, Amplatz stiff guidewire) is advanced into the duodenum. The track is then coaxially dilated with rigid Teflon dilators. On occasion, a tight biliary stricture may require additional dilation with a high-pressure angioplasty balloon to facilitate placement of a drainage catheter. At initial entry, an 8 Fr internal–external biliary catheter is left in place through the obstructing lesion into the duodenum, with side holes placed proximally and distally to the obstruction. The Ring biliary catheter (Cook) or Cope loop self-retaining catheter (Cook, or Medi-tech) is most commonly chosen, as either provides a sufficient drainage lumen and resistance to dislodgement. Afterwards, limited catheter cholangiography is performed to confirm appropriate position of the catheter and drainage holes. The catheter is sutured securely to the skin, and a collection bag is attached for gravity drainage of the bile (Fig. 29-2).

If there is evidence of hemobilia upon initial catheter insertion, repeated irrigation with small aliquots of sterile saline is appropriate for the first 24 h after tube placement to assure catheter patency. Sterile saline (5 cc) is injected into the catheter, and the catheter is allowed to drain passively. Suction on the catheter may aspirate duodenal contents into the liver, increasing the risk of sepsis.

Occasionally, a high-grade biliary stricture cannot be traversed at the initial session. In this case, a catheter is placed above the obstruction and left to external drainage. Usually after a 2- to 3-day period of external drainage, more difficult strictures can be traversed, allowing placement of an internal–external catheter.

In patients requiring long-term drainage, after a period of decompression, the initial drainage catheter is enlarged to at least 10 Fr. The external portion of the tube can then be capped, resulting in internal biliary drainage into the duodenum. The Cope catheter with a self-retaining loop is recommended, and the retention loop is placed in the duodenum, creating a stable catheter position for long-term drainage.

Long-term external biliary drainage is usually avoided because of the risk of dehydration and electrolyte depletion. Insertion of an

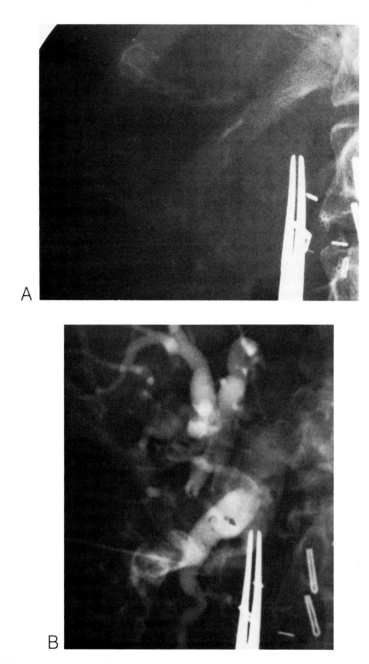

Fig. 29-2. (A) In anticipation of percutaneous drainage the area of the porta hepatis is marked with a hemostat. **(B)** A 22-gauge needle is used to enter and opacify the dilated biliary ductal system. (*Figure continues.*)

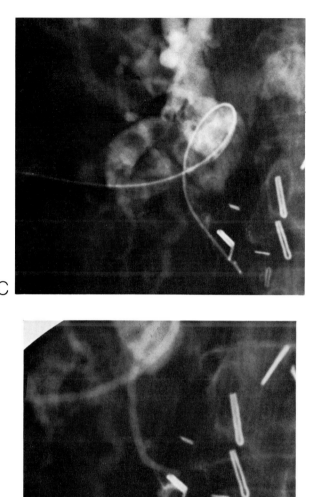

C

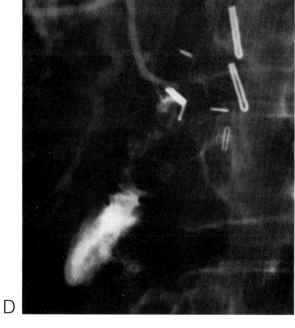

D

Fig. 29-2. (*Continued*). **(C)** A 0.035-in. guidewire is placed in a stable position within the ducts using a one-stick system. **(D)** A catheter is advanced into the ductal system and used to negotiate a wire through a strictured choledochoenteric anastamosis. (*Figure continues.*)

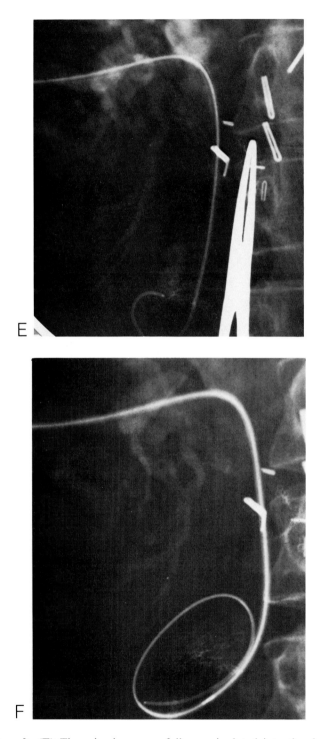

Fig. 29-2. (*Continued*). **(E)** The wire is successfully manipulated into the duodenum, and initial dilatation of the stricture is performed. **(F)** The flexible guidewire is replaced with a stiffer exchange wire, the flexible tip of which is coiled within the duodenum. (*Figure continues.*)

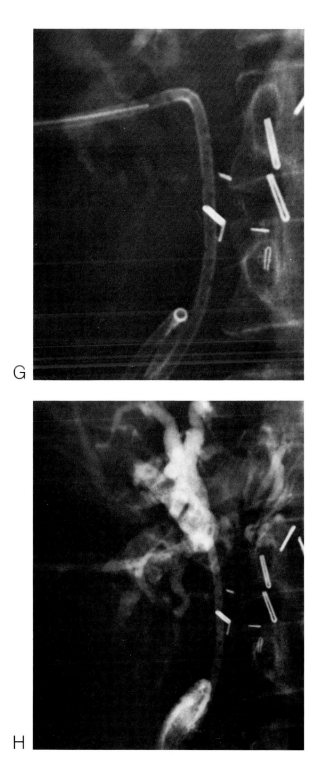

G

H

Fig. 29-2. (*Continued*). **(G)** A Cope loop biliary catheter is placed with holes proximal and distal to the stricture. The most proximal hole is identified with a guidewire to assure an intraductal location. **(H)** Contrast injection confirms an appropriate catheter position with filling of the intrahepatic biliary ducts.

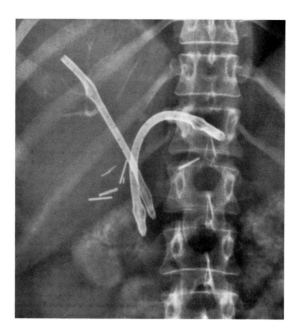

Fig. 29-3. Left- and right-sided biliary endoprostheses have been placed for high hepatic duct strictures. Mushroom-type retention devices above and below the stricture prevent prosthesis migration.

internal–external catheter reestablishes antegrade bile flow and reduces the chances of catheter dislodgement.

BILIARY ENDOPROSTHESES

Indications: Endoprostheses (completely internalized biliary stents) are also employed for palliation of malignant biliary obstruction. The advantages of an endoprosthesis rather than an internal–external drainage catheter include elimination of entry-site pain, skin irritation, and the need for regular catheter care. The absence of an external catheter segment to serve as a constant reminder to the patient of his underlying malignancy may improve the patient's psychological well-being. The main disadvantage is that if the endoprosthesis malfunctions and cannot be exchanged endoscopically, then repeat percutaneous transhepatic biliary drainage may be required.

TYPES OF ENDOPROSTHESES

Plastic endoprostheses consist of tapered-tipped segments of polymeric catheter material that can be loaded onto a stiffening cannula for over-the-wire insertion. Plastic endoprostheses are available in a variety of materials and also vary in caliber, length, side-hole size and configuration, and presence or absence of retention devices (Fig. 29-3).

A variety of newer expandable metallic endoprostheses are available for use in the biliary tract. Examples include the modified Gianturco stent (Cook, Bloomington, IN), the Wallstent (Schneider, Minneapolis, MN), and the Palmaz stent (Johnson & Johnson, Warren, NJ). These metallic stents are deliverable through 7 to 10 Fr introducer sheaths and are either self-expanding or balloon expandable.

TECHNIQUE FOR INSERTION OF PLASTIC ENDOPROSTHESES

Although it may be technically feasible to insert an endoprosthesis at the time of initial percutaneous transhepatic biliary drainage, to reduce patient discomfort and risk the procedure is usually performed in two separate steps at least a few days apart.

Following an initial catheter cholangiogram, the existing internal–external catheter is removed over a heavy-duty guidewire positioned with its tip well into the duodenum. The endoprosthesis and an accompanying pusher are loaded onto a stiffening cannula. The track is dilated with rigid coaxial dilators or a high-pressure angioplasty balloon, and the endoprosthesis, stiffening cannula, and pusher are inserted over the guidewire and advanced as a unit into the appropriate position. A peel-away sheath with a luminal diameter large enough to accept the endoprosthesis may be necessary to facilitate placement. Once the stiffening cannula is removed, contrast material can be injected through the nontapered pusher with the aid of a side arm adapter to assure correct endoprosthesis position. The pusher is then exchanged for a slightly smaller external drainage catheter, which is left in place pending follow-up cholangiography to assess stent patency.

The location and nature of the obstructing lesion determine whether the endoprosthesis needs to extend into the duodenum.

When endoprostheses placed in an antegrade fashion malfunction because of either occlusion or migration, endoscopic manipulation may be technically feasible. If not, a variety of percutaneous techniques for endoprosthesis repositioning, disimpaction, and exchange have been described. The details of these manipulations are beyond the scope of this handbook.

SUGGESTED READINGS

Günther RW, Schild H, Thelen M: Review article: percutaneous transhepatic biliary drainage: experience with 311 procedures. Cardiovasc Intervent Radiol 11:65, 1988

Harbin WP, Mueller PR, Ferrucci JT Jr: Transhepatic cholangiography: complications and use patterns of the fine-needle technique. Radiology 135:15, 1980

Lammer J: Biliary endoprostheses: plastic versus metal stents. Radiol Clin North Am 28:1211, 1990

McLean GK, Burke DR: Role of endoprostheses in the management of malignant biliary obstruction. Radiology 170:961, 1989

Mueller PR, vanSonnenberg E, Ferrucci JT Jr: Percutaneous biliary drainage: technical and catheter-related problems in 200 procedures. AJR 138:17, 1982

30

Percutaneous Urinary Intervention

Ronald J. Zagoria

ANTEGRADE PYELOGRAPHY AND WHITAKER TESTING

Antegrade Pyelography Indications: Antegrade pyelography is performed for the opacification of the pelvocalyceal system and ureter in patients with contraindications to intravascular contrast material administration. It may also be performed as a prelude to nephrostomy drainage or Whitaker testing.

Whitaker Test Indications: Whitaker testing is performed for objective evaluation and quantification of the urodynamic significance of suspected urinary tract obstruction.

Risks: Both antegrade pyelography and the Whitaker test require fine-needle puncture of the renal collecting system, with a small associated risk of vascular injury or sepsis. Contraindications include coagulopathy and active urinary infection, which should be assessed and corrected prior to this procedure. Because vascular fields are transgressed, there is also risk of reaction to contrast material.

Pyelography Technique: A broad-spectrum antibiotic (usually a cephalosporin), is administered prior to the procedure and every 8 h while the patient is hospitalized for up to 48 h after the procedure. If no drainage catheter is placed, antibiotics can be discontinued after the diagnostic procedure. The bladder should be catheterized before the patient is placed in prone position on the fluoroscopy table. The flank is cleansed and draped using standard sterile techniques. The kidney location is established with fluoroscopy or ultrasonography. An abdominal radiograph is often useful in identifying renal position. If the kidney is not visible, a puncture site is initially

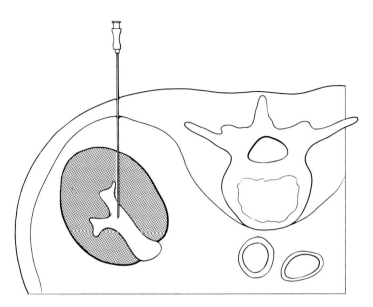

Fig. 30-1. The renal collecting system is accessed using a vertical puncture from a direct posterior approach with a 21- or 22-gauge needle for antegrade pyelography or as a prelude to other interventions.

selected empirically 2 to 3 cm lateral to the top of the L2 vertebral body. The area of planned puncture is anesthetized with 1% lidocaine. A vertical puncture is made with a 21- or 22-gauge thin-walled needle at the desired site while the patient suspends respiration (Fig. 30-1).

The stylet is removed and a syringe attached. Continuous aspiration is performed as the needle is gradually withdrawn. When aspiration returns urine, withdrawal is halted. This urine aspirate is saved for culture. A small amount of intermediate iodine concentration contrast material (300 mg I/ml) is injected to confirm satisfactory needle position. Contrast material should flow freely away from the needle tip. Once a satisfactory position is confirmed, the collecting system and ureter are opacified with injection of additional contrast material under intermittent fluoroscopic monitoring. Overdistention of the collecting system should be avoided to reduce the risk of sepsis. Spot films are obtained as needed to demonstrate the entire pelvocalyceal system, ureter, and sites of suspected pathology.

Whitaker Test Technique: The Whitaker test is performed by placing a needle into the collecting system in the same manner as described for antegrade pyelography. With the needle in place, the bladder is emptied, and manometers, infusion lines, infusion pump, and bladder drainage conduit are connected as shown (Fig. 30-2). The bladder and renal pelvis pressures are measured immediately prior to the start of infusion and immediately after each timed infusion volume. Dilute contrast material is infused at a rate of 5 ml/min for 10 min. After pressures are recorded, infusion is repeated at a rate of 10 ml/min for 10 min and, finally, at a rate of 15 ml/min for 10 min. The test is discontinued if renal pelvis pressure exceeds 40 cm of water. If the results are normal or equivocal, the test is repeated after the bladder fills.

The patient should be instructed to notify personnel if symptoms are reproduced during the infusion. The reproduction of symptoms further supports the presence of urodynamically significant obstruction.

Interpretation of Results

Renal pelvic pressure minus bladder pressure	Interpretation
<13 cm H_2O	normal
13–22 cm H_2O	mild or equivocal obstruction
23–40 cm H_2O	moderate ureteral obstruction
>40 cm H_2O	severe obstruction

PERCUTANEOUS NEPHROSTOMY DRAINAGE

Indications: Nephrostomy drainage is used for the relief of urinary tract obstruction, urine diversion for treatment of urinary tract fistula or perforation, decompression of an infected urinary tract, or as a prelude to additional urinary tract interventions.

Risks: Risks of the procedure include septicemia (2%), life-threatening vascular injury (1% to 2%), and adjacent organ injury (< 1%). The only absolute contraindication is the presence of an uncorrected bleeding diathesis.

Technique: When possible, the patient should be interviewed prior to the procedure and informed consent should be obtained. Antibiotics should be initiated prior to attempted percutaneous nephrostomy drainage. Culture-specific antibiotics are preferred for patients with known urinary tract infections. If no infection is suspected, a broad-spectrum cephalosporin is given intravenously immediately before the procedure and every 8 h, for up to 48 h while the patient remains hospitalized. With a bladder catheter in place, the patient should be placed in prone position on the fluoroscopic table. The target renal collecting system is then opacified. This can be achieved with antegrade pyelography techniques as described in the previous section, with the injection of intravenous contrast material, or with retrograde injection of contrast material through a ureteral stent or urinary conduit. An intermediate iodine concentration contrast material is used.

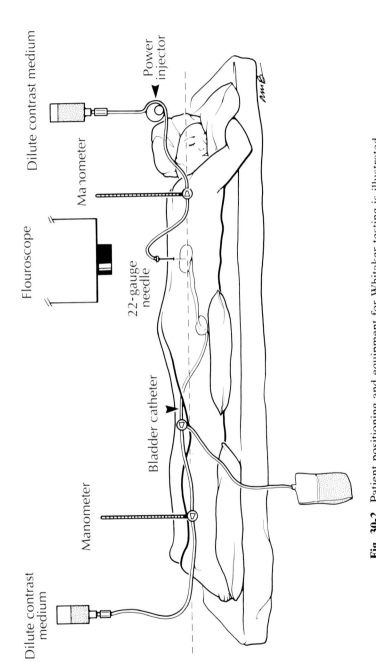

Fig. 30-2. Patient positioning and equipment for Whitaker testing is illustrated.

Dilute contrast medium

Power injector

Manometer

Flouroscope

22-gauge needle

Bladder catheter

Manometer

Dilute contrast medium

Overdistention should be avoided. After partial opacification of the collecting system, 2 to 10 cc of room air can be injected to aid in identification of the posterior calyces. A posterior calyx, preferably below the 12th rib, is selected for definitive puncture. Once the appropriate calyx to be punctured is identified, the fluoroscopy tube is rotated 25° from the vertical position, ipsilateral to the side of entry. Alternatively, the patient's flank can be elevated 25° when vertical fluoroscopy is employed. The puncture site is identified by fluoroscopic localization of the area of skin directly over the planned site of calyceal entry. This area of skin is then anesthetized with 1% lidocaine without epinephrine. Both superficial and deep skin anesthetization should be performed prior to calyceal puncture. A small skin nick is made with a scalpel at the site of skin puncture. The calyx is then punctured with 22- to 18-gauge needle under continuous fluoroscopic monitoring while the patient suspends respiration (Fig. 30-3A). A radiolucent needle holder is useful during this step to allow needle guidance while the operator's hands remain outside the fluoroscopy field.

Once the calyx is punctured, urine is aspirated to confirm a position within the collecting system. An appropriately sized guidewire is then advanced into the collecting system. The needle is removed and an angiographic catheter is advanced over the guidewire to manipulate it into a stable position (Fig. 30-3B). The catheter is then removed and the track is dilated over the guidewire to an appropriate size for nephrostomy tube placement (Fig. 30-3C).

For simple urine drainage, an 8 to 10 Fr tube is adequate. For a solitary kidney or in patients with pyonephrosis, 12 to 14 Fr tubes are recommended. Only self-retaining nephrostomy tubes should be used. The Cope loop drainage catheters provide sufficient retention capability and drainage caliber in most circumstances (Fig. 30-3D). Prior to termination of the procedure, contrast material is injected through the nephrostomy tube to confirm satisfactory position and function of the tube.

The patient should be visited daily for 3 days following nephrostomy tube placement to ensure adequate tube function. Urine output should be monitored carefully while the patient is hospitalized. Hematuria is routine for up to 72 h following nephrostomy tube placement. The nephrostomy tube should routinely be changed every 4 to 8 weeks to prevent tube occlusion.

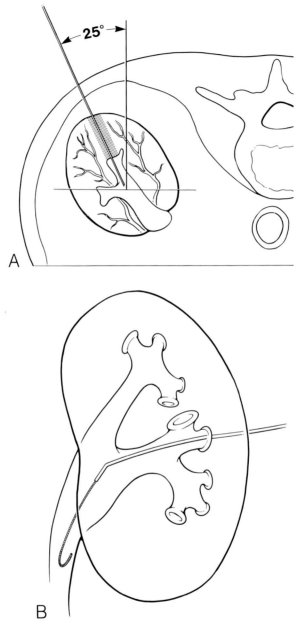

Fig. 30-3. (A) A 25° posterior oblique approach is used for puncture of the renal collecting system when the track will be subsequently dilated. This approach avoids the major renal artery branches. **(B)** Following puncture, a guidewire is manipulated into the ureter using an angled angiographic catheter. (*Figure continues.*)

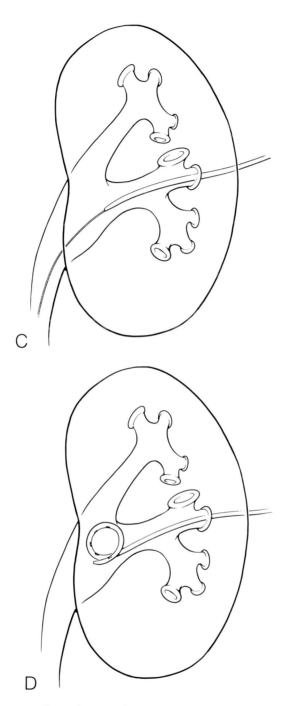

Fig. 30-3 (*Continued*). **(C)** A dilator is passed over the guidewire to enlarge the track prior to nephrostomy tube placement. **(D)** A Cope loop nephrostomy catheter is positioned in the renal pelvis.

LARGE-BORE NEPHROSTOMY TRACK-CREATION

Indications: Large-bore nephrostomy entry is usually created for endoscopy with a rigid or large-bore flexible endoscope, including those required for percutaneous nephrolithotomy. In addition, large-bore tracks may be required for more complicated interventions such as ureteral occlusion. Percutaneous stone removal procedures are preferred to other techniques when renal stones are large (>25 mm), are branched in configuration, are composed of cystine, or are associated with ureteral obstruction. A patient may exceed the weight limitations of a lithotripsy device, or in some cases complete and immediate stone removal may be essential.

Risks: Risks of large-bore nephrostomy track creation include renal hemorrhage necessitating blood transfusion (up to 10%), sepsis (2%), and adjacent organ injury (1%). The only absolute contraindication is the presence of an uncorrected bleeding diathesis. If rigid nephroscopy is planned, a skin-to-calyx distance less than 18 cm is essential. Flexible endoscopy can be performed over a greater distance through a nephrostomy track that has been allowed to mature.

Technique: When possible, the physician performing the procedure should interview the patient, explain the procedure, and obtain informed consent. A broad-spectrum antibiotic is administered intravenously prior to initiating the procedure and is continued after the procedure while the patient remains hospitalized.

With the patient in prone position, the flank is cleansed and draped in a sterile fashion. The renal collecting system is opacified using the same techniques described in the percutaneous nephrostomy drainage section. A posterior calyx that gives access to the desired segment of the urinary system should be selected. For nephrolithotomy, the selected calyx should allow the greatest access to the stone. If the ureter is the main focus of interest, a mid- or upper-pole calyx should be selected. Because of increased risks and greater patient discomfort, an intercostal approach should be avoided if possible.

Following the steps outlined in the section on percutaneous nephrostomy drainage, the selected calyx is punctured. Once the calyx is punctured, urine is aspirated to confirm position. An appropriately sized guidewire is then advanced into the collecting system. With large stones, the guidewire must be advanced around the stone; this task may require redirection with a curved catheter and guidewires of varying flexibility. Once a guidewire with a 0.035-in. diameter or greater is advanced into a stable position, ideally within the ureter, the nephrostomy tract is dilated to 9 Fr. The next dilatation step is performed with a dilator/sheath introducer, which is advanced well into the pelvocalyceal system. The dilator is removed, and at least one additional guidewire is advanced into a secure position through the sheath (Fig. 30-4A). This guidewire will serve as a safety wire during the remainder of the procedure.

A high-pressure balloon dilatation catheter is then advanced over one of the guidewires for further track dilatation. The inflated balloon diameter should be 10 mm (30 Fr), and the balloon length should be adequate to dilate the entire nephrostomy track with one or two balloon inflations. The balloon is then inflated to its maximum capacity (Fig. 30-4B). If balloon dilatation is incomplete, rigid coaxial dilators can be employed to complete the dilatation.

Following dilatation of the track, a 30 Fr diameter sheath is advanced into the pelvocalyceal system (Fig. 30-4C). Endoscopy can be performed through this sheath immediately, or a drainage catheter can be passed through the sheath if endoscopy is deferred. Once a large-bore nephrostomy catheter is placed through the track, a 5 Fr catheter should be advanced over the safety wire until its tip is in a stable position, preferably within the bladder. Contrast material should be injected through the large-bore nephrostomy tube to confirm satisfactory position and function of the tube. The guidewire is then removed, and both nephrostomy catheters are sutured to the skin.

The patient should be visited daily for at least 3 days to assess tube function and the possibility of nephrostomy complications. Urine output should be monitored carefully. Hematuria routinely lasts for up to 72 h following nephrostomy tube placement. If tubes are to be left in place for a prolonged period, they should be changed every 6 to 8 weeks.

URETERAL STENTING

Indications: Ureteral stents are placed for the maintenance of ureteral patency in patients with stones, strictures, and malignancies. In addition, these stents are placed as a mechanical aid to enhance healing in patients with ureteral fistulas or perforations, or following ureteral dilatation.

Risks: Antegrade ureteral stent placement is a very safe procedure. The major risks with this procedure are those associated with percutaneous nephrostomy track creation, which is done prior to stenting. Transient hematuria is a universal sequela of ureteral stent placement. Significant hemorrhage is rarely associated with stent place-

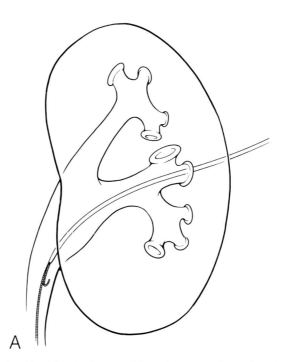

A

Fig. 30-4. (A) A second "safety" guidewire is passed into the ureter through a sheath. Safety wires should be employed prior to any interventional urinary tract procedure more complex than simple nephrostomy drainage. (*Figure continues.*)

Technique:

ment. Septicemia can occur following ureteral stenting but is quite rare in a decompressed renal unit. Ureteral perforation occurs occasionally during attempted ureteral stent placement. Although perforation may interfere with further progress in placing a ureteral stent, it is of little clinical significance if adequate renal drainage is provided.

Percutaneous nephrostomy drainage should be accomplished as previously described. If stent placement is anticipated after nephrostomy drainage is established, a midpole or upper calyx should be selected to provide the most favorable approach to the ureter.

Initially, a nephrostogram is obtained using intermediate iodine concentration contrast material. The ureteropelvic junction should be visualized to guide catheterization. After the nephrostomy tube is removed over a guidewire, angiographic techniques are used to manipulate a catheter through the ureteropelvic junction and into the bladder. The correct stent length is then determined with the bent guidewire technique. The catheter tip is placed in the bladder, and a guidewire is advanced so that its tip is within the catheter just below the ureterovesical junction. The guidewire

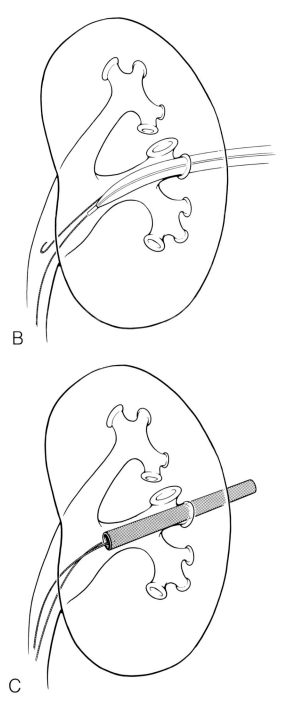

B

C

Fig. 30-4 (*Continued*). **(B)** Rapid track dilatation is obtained by inflation of a balloon catheter that has been advanced over the ''working'' guidewire. **(C)** A large-bore sheath has been placed following track dilatation in anticipation of renal endoscopy.

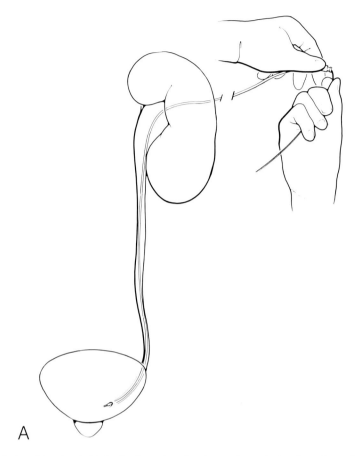

A

Fig. 30-5. (A) A guidewire is kinked where it exits the catheter hub when the guidewire tip is at the ureterovesical junction. This is the first step in determining the correct length of the stent to be placed. (*Figure continues.*)

is kinked at the exit of the catheter hub at the flank (Fig. 30-5A). The guidewire is then retracted until its tip is in the renal pelvis within the catheter. A second kink is made where the guidewire exits the catheter hub at the flank (Fig. 30-5B). The guidewire is then completely removed, leaving the catheter in place. The distance between the two guidewire kinks is an exact measure of the distance between the ureteropelvic and ureterovesical junction. This measurement determines the length of the straight segment of the ureteral stent between the retention coils.

A stiff guidewire is then advanced through the catheter and the flexible end coiled within the bladder. The catheter is removed. A tapered 8 Fr angiographic catheter is then advanced over the guidewire into the bladder. If no resistance is encountered, an 8 Fr or smaller stent can be placed subsequent to catheter removal.

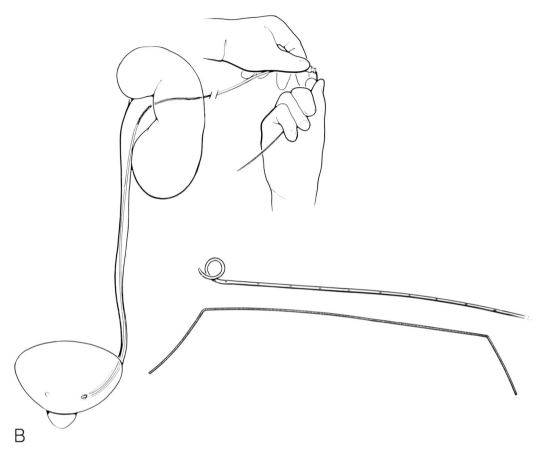

B

Fig. 30-5 (*Continued*). **(B)** The guidewire is again kinked at its exit from the catheter hub when the tip of the guidewire is in the renal pelvis. The distance between the kinks determines stent length or extent of holes to be made in a customized internal/external stent. (*Figure continues.*)

If resistance is encountered, the 8 Fr catheter is removed and replaced with a 9 Fr ureteral introducer sheath (Cook, Blooming-ton, IN). This sheath should be advanced into the bladder or as far as possible into the ureter. With either of these techniques, the pusher that is provided is used to advance the stent over the guidewire until its tip is well within the bladder. If marked resistance is encountered, balloon dilatation of the stenotic portion of the ureter may facilitate further stent advancement.

After advancing an adequate length of stent into the bladder, the guidewire is retracted to reconstitute the coil in the lower end of the stent. Fluoroscopy of the renal end of the stent is then performed to ascertain whether the remaining length of stent is adequate to allow for reconstitution of the upper loop within the renal pelvis. If the stent has been advanced too far distally, it can be

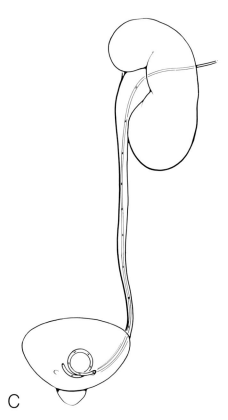

C

Fig. 30 (*Continued*). **(C)** An internal/external stent has been placed with its lower end looped in the bladder and drainage holes along its length within the ureter and renal pelvis as determined using the bent guidewire technique. These holes will allow for either internal or external urine drainage.

retracted an appropriate distance by means of a suture that is supplied with the stent. The suture is woven through two holes in the upper end of the stent.

Prior to final placement of the stent, the introducer sheath, if employed, is removed. The retracting suture is removed while maintaining stent position with gentle forward pressure on the pusher. The guidewire is then withdrawn further so that only the flexible portion of the guidewire remains within the proximal ureteral stent. The pusher is then used to advance the stent through the remaining segment of the nephrostomy track and into the renal pelvis while the wire is simultaneously withdrawn. This technique allows the upper end to form a loop configuration.

Once the upper end of the stent forms, a guidewire can be replaced into the renal pelvis via the pusher catheter. A nephrostomy tube can be placed over this wire or over a safety guidewire if one has been inserted prior to stent positioning. If significant hematuria is present, the nephrostomy tube should be left open to external drainage until the urine clears to prevent occlusion of the ureteral stent because of bleeding. Once the urine is clear, the nephrostomy tube can be capped or clamped to force internal drainage of urine through the stent. If minimal or no hematuria complicates stent placement, the nephrostomy tube can be capped immediately following the procedure. The nephrostomy tube should be left in place for approximately 24 h. If no symptoms of ureteral occlusion develop, the nephrostomy tube can be removed under fluoroscopic guidance after a nephrostogram demonstrates satisfactory position and function of the ureteral stent. Fluoroscopy is used to ensure that the renal stent is not dislodged while the nephrostomy tube is removed.

An alternative method of stenting is the placement of an internal/external ureteral stent. This technique employs a single catheter extending from the patient's flank through the kidney into the bladder. This catheter should be used when ureteral stenting is indicated but prolonged percutaneous renal access is desired. Placement of these stents closely parallels placement of internal ureteral stents. The bent wire technique is used to determine the site of holes to be placed in the catheter for drainage (Fig. 30-5). While ready-made catheters of this variety are available, internal/external stents can be tailor-made by modifying extended length Cope loop nephrostomy catheters. Modification of these catheters simply entails fashioning side holes along the desired length of the catheter shaft (Fig. 30-5B & C).

Long-term care of patients with internal ureteral stents is assumed by urologists. These stents are periodically changed or removed at cystoscopy. Internal/external ureteral stents should also be changed periodically (every 6 to 8 weeks) to avoid stent occlusion. While in place, these stents can be maintained either with external bag drainage or with external capping, which forces internal drainage into the bladder.

SUGGESTED READINGS

Lang EK: Percutaneous nephrostolithotomy and lithotripsy: a multi-institutional survey of complications. Radiology 162:25, 1987

Pfister RC, Newhouse JH, Hendren WH: Percutaneous pyelouretal urodynamics. Urol Clin North Am 9:41, 1982

31

Drugs Used in Vascular and Interventional Radiology

William P. Jones
Ray Dyer

Drugs in the amnestic, analgesic, and antibiotic classes are routinely used in the performance of vascular and interventional radiology in adults. In addition, a working knowledge of a few additional drugs in the vasodilator, vasoconstrictor, and anticoagulant classes will extend the diagnostic and therapeutic usefulness of angiography and may help to prevent procedural complications.

VASODILATORS

Tolazoline hydrochloride (Priscoline) is a vasodilator that acts directly on vascular smooth muscle. The vasodilatory effect may be useful in the demonstration of peripheral vessels during extremity angiography, may improve flow from the arterial to the venous vascular beds for increased mesenteric or portal venous opacification, may provide prophylaxis and therapy of catheter- or guidewire-induced vasospasm, and may be useful in the assessment of the hemodynamic significance of an arterial stenosis.

Tolazoline is supplied in vials containing 100 mg/4 cc. For injection via the arterial catheter into the vascular field to be evaluated, 25 mg of tolazoline is diluted in 5 to 10 cc of sterile saline. Maximal vasodilatation occurs 20 to 30 s after injection. Contrast material volumes for diagnostic angiography should be increased in response to the vasodilatory effect. The same dose of tolazoline can be given via the catheter to prevent or treat catheter- or guidewire-induced vasospasm. In the assessment of the hemodynamic significance of an arterial stenosis, 25 mg of tolazoline is delivered distal to the arterial stenosis (which simulates the increased vascular demand of exercise in the distal vessels) and arterial pressures are obtained distal and proximal to the lesion after 30 to 60 s.

At the dose used for diagnostic angiography, the risk associated with tolazoline is minor. Transient hypotension, which is readily responsive to fluid resuscitation and leg elevation, may be seen. Tachycardia and cardiac arrhythmias may occur. The drug should be used with care in patients with known coronary artery disease.

Nitroglycerin is a direct smooth muscle dilator that may be used for improved opacification of small vessel beds during diagnostic angiography (especially in the distal extremities) and in the treatment of catheter- or guidewire-induced vasospasm.

Injectable nitroglycerin is available in vials containing up to 100 mg of nitroglycerin. For intraarterial use, the usual dose is 100 μg. Nitroglycerin should be diluted in normal saline to provide 100 μg/5 cc. The onset of the vasodilatory effect after intraarterial injection is rapid. Diagnostic angiography should be performed within 15 to 30 s after injection. Multiple doses, up to 300 to 500 μg, may be given for the treatment of vasospasm.

Hypotension with reflex tachycardia may develop, and thus nitroglycerin should not be used in patients with profound hypotension or uncorrected hypovolemia. Drug-induced hypotension is usually responsive to fluid resuscitation and leg elevation.

Papaverine hydrochloride is a direct smooth muscle relaxant with resultant vasodilatory effects. Traditionally, papaverine has been used in infusion therapy for mesenteric ischemia (see Ch. 12). More recently, papaverine has been used for intracavernosal injection (often in combination with other drugs) for evaluation and therapy of vasculogenic impotence.

Papaverine is supplied in vials containing 60 mg/2 cc. For therapy of nonocclusive mesenteric ischemia, diagnostic angiography is performed after selective placement of a superior mesenteric artery catheter. If nonocclusive ischemia is suspected, a papaverine infusion of 3 mg/min is given for 20 min. Following this initial infusion, a 30-mg papaverine bolus is given and arteriography is repeated. If improved flow is seen, infusion can be continued at a rate of 0.75 mg/min. Infusion may be continued for up to 24 h, as therapy to improve cardiac output and reduce peripheral vasoconstriction is ongoing, or up to the time of surgery to protect underperfused bowel. Improvement in the degree of vasoconstriction seen angiographically does not rule out significant ischemic bowel injury, but failure of response to papaverine strongly suggests bowel infarction.

Risks of drug administration include hypotension, abdominal discomfort, and diarrhea.

Nifedipine (Procardia) is a calcium channel blocking agent that produces relaxation of arterial smooth muscle. It is commonly used as a prophylactic agent to prevent vascular spasm induced by catheters and guidewires during angioplasty.

Nifedipine is supplied as a 10-mg capsule for oral administration. It is rapidly absorbed by the sublingual route, and can be delivered in this manner by puncturing the capsule with a needle and squeezing the liquid contents beneath the patient's tongue. The capsule is then swallowed. Onset of the pharmacologic effect after a sublingual dose occurs in 10 to 15 min, which allows administration immediately prior to the angiographic procedure.

Nifedipine can cause hypotension and reflex tachycardia, which may precipitate an attack of angina pectoris. Patients receiving other calcium channel blocking agents (verapamil) in their medical regimen obtain no increased benefit with nifedipine.

VASOCONSTRICTORS

Epinephrine produces vasoconstriction in many vascular beds, but especially in the precapillary beds of the kidney. Normal renal vessels are constricted in response to intraarterial epinephrine, while tumor vessels, which lack ordered smooth muscle cells, fail to constrict. This effect enhances flow into the tumor vessels because of their lack of response. Renal arterial injection of epinephrine with reduction of arterial flow will enhance the opacification of the renal venous bed during the performance of renal venography.

Epinephrine is supplied in many different concentrations, but those usually available for injection include the 1 mg/cc (1 : 1,000 dilution) or 1 mg/10 cc (1 : 10,000 dilution). For intraarterial use, 0.5 mg is diluted in 500 cc of normal saline to yield a solution of 1 μg/cc. For enhancement of tumor vascularity in the renal arterial bed, 3 to 6 μg of epinephrine is injected via the selective renal artery catheter over 20 to 30 s followed by angiography with a reduced volume of contrast material. For augmentation of renal venography, 6 to 10 μg of epinephrine is injected via the renal arterial catheter to slow arterial flow, and venography is performed through the renal venous catheter.

At doses used for diagnostic angiography, systemic effects of epinephrine are negligible. However, care should be taken in patients with a history of angina pectoris and coronary artery disease.

Vasopressin (*Pitressin*) produces marked splanchnic vasoconstriction and is useful in the control of gastrointestinal bleeding, especially for gastric mucosal and colonic diverticular sources. Bleeding from peptic ulceration at gastroduodenal or anastomotic sites may not respond as well.

Vasopressin is supplied in vials containing 20 units/cc. After identification of a bleeding site, the angiographic catheter is advanced as selectively as possible into the source artery. Next, 100 units of vasopressin are diluted in 250 cc of normal saline, yielding 0.4 units/cc. Initial infusion is begun at 0.2 units/min (30 cc/h) for 20 min. A repeat arteriogram is performed to assess response. If no response is seen, infusion is increased to 0.4 units/min (60 cc/h), and the angiogram is repeated after 20 min. Infusion rates in excess of 0.4 units/min provide no increased hemostatic efficacy and increase the risk of side effects of infusion. The infusion can be continued prior to surgery, or the dose can be halved every 12 h until the patient can be weaned. Prior to catheter removal, an infusion of normal saline for 12 h should be performed through the selective catheter to assure there is no recurrence of bleeding.

Vasopressin should be used with care in patients with coronary artery disease, as vasoconstriction may precipitate angina pectoris and myocardial infarction. Cardiac arrhythmias, especially bradycardia, may also develop. The antidiuretic effect of vasopressin may cause electrolyte disturbances and fluid retention. Muscular and abdominal cramps, nausea, and bronchial constriction are additional side effects that may occur. Because of these effects, a patient receiving a vasopressin infusion should be monitored in a high nurse-to-patient ratio care setting.

ANTICOAGULANTS

Heparin where given intravascularly combines with antithrombin III, which results in the inactivation of thrombin. As a result, conversion of fibrinogen to fibrin is blocked. Heparin should be administered when there is risk of thrombosis during a vascular or interventional procedure, as in the performance of transluminal angioplasty, or when a catheter traverses a narrowed vessel significantly impeding antegrade blood flow. Heparin may also be used in flush solutions to prevent catheter thrombosis.

Heparin in a concentration of 2,000 units/cc is most useful in angiography. For the prevention of pericatheter or periprocedural thrombosis, a bolus of 50 to 100 units/kg (2,000 to 5,000 units for an average adult) can be given intraarterially. To prevent catheter thrombosis, 2 to 4 units of heparin can be added per cc of flush solution.

The half-life of heparin varies with the administered dose and is prolonged in patients with renal and hepatic dysfunction. In the normal patient, at doses used for angiography, the half-life is 45 to 90 min. The effects of heparin can be reversed with protamine sulfate. One milligram of protamine will reverse the effect of 100 units of heparin. The dose of protamine should be adjusted to account for normal heparin elimination.

With the doses used for angiography, side effects primarily relate to bleeding complications at the catheter entry site. These complications can usually be controlled with manual compression and heparin reversal as needed.

SUGGESTED READINGS

Abrams HL: The response of neoplastic renal vessels to epinephrine in man. Radiology 82:217, 1964

Baum S, Nusbaum M: The control of gastrointestinal hemorrhage by selective mesenteric arterial infusion of vasopressin. Radiology 98:497, 1971

Becker GJ, Katzen BT, Dake MD: Noncoronary angioplasty. Radiology 170:921, 1989

Clark RA, Colley DP: Pharmacoangiography: techniques and clinical uses. Radiographics 1:43, 1981

Gilman AG, Rall TW, Nies AS, Taylor P (eds): The Pharmacologic Basis of Therapeutics. 8th Ed. Pergamon Press, New York, 1990

Miller DL: Heparin in angiography: current patterns of use. Radiology 172:1007, 1989

Olin TB, Reuter SR: A pharmacoangiographic method for improving nephrophlebography. Radiology 85:1036, 1965

Reuter SR, Redman HC, Cho KJ: Gastrointestinal Angiography. 3rd Ed. WB Saunders, Philadelphia, 1986

Siegelman SS, Sprayregen S, Boley JJ: Angiographic diagnosis of mesenteric arterial vasoconstriction. Radiology 112:533, 1974

Index

Page numbers followed by an *f* indicate figures, and those followed by a *t* indicate tables.